PATTERNS OF PRACTICE

by the same author

Keepers of the Soul
The Five Guardian Elements of Acupuncture
ISBN 978 1 84819 185 3
eISBN 978 0 85701 146 6

The Simple Guide to Five Element Acupuncture
ISBN 978 1 84819 186 0
eISBN 978 0 85701 147 3

The Handbook of Five Element Practice
ISBN 978 1 84819 188 4
eISBN 978 0 85701 145 9

MASTERING THE ART OF FIVE ELEMENT ACUPUNCTURE

PATTERNS OF PRACTICE

NORA FRANGLEN

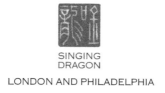

SINGING
DRAGON

LONDON AND PHILADELPHIA

Quote on page 6 from *Life and Fate* by Vasily Grossman, published by Harvill Press, reprinted by permission of The Random House Group Limited. Afterword reprinted by kind permission of the Maryland University of Integrative Health, Maryland, USA, formerly the Tai Sophia Institute, www.muih.edu.

This edition published in 2014
by Singing Dragon
an imprint of Jessica Kingsley Publishers
73 Collier Street
London N1 9BE, UK
and
400 Market Street, Suite 400
Philadelphia, PA 19106, USA

www.singingdragon.com

First edition published by the School of Five Element Acupuncture, 2009

Library of Congress Cataloging in Publication Data
Franglen, Nora.
  [Pattern of things]
  Patterns of practice : mastering the art of five
element acupuncture / Nora Franglen.
      pages cm
  Originally published as: The pattern of things : viewing
life through the prism of the five elements.
London : School of Five Element Acupuncture, 2009.
  Includes bibliographical references.
  ISBN 978-1-84819-187-7 (alk. paper)
  1. Acupuncture. 2. Five agents (Chinese philosophy) I. Title.
  RM184.F58625 2014
  615.8'92--dc23
                                            2013024598

British Library Cataloguing in Publication Data
A CIP catalogue record for this book is available from the British Library

ISBN 978 1 84819 187 7
eISBN 978 0 85701 148 0

Printed and bound in Great Britain

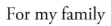
For my family

'It was the very strangest of feelings, something you could never share with any other person – not even your wife, your mother, your brother, your son, your friend or your father. It was the secret of your soul. However passionately it might long to, your soul could never betray this secret. You carry away this sense of your life without having ever shared it with anyone: the miracle of a particular individual whose conscious and unconscious contain everything good and bad, everything funny, sweet, shameful, pitiful, timid, tender, uncertain, that has happened from childhood to old age – fused into the mysterious sense of an individual life.'

Vasily Grossman, Life and Fate

CONTENTS

ABOUT THE AUTHOR 9

Introduction 11

1. Challenges of a Five Element Practice: Listening Palace 17

2. The Imprint of Imbalance: Penetrating Inside 27

3. The Otherness of Others: Assembly of Ancestors 35

4. Doorways to the Elements: Spirit Path 43

5. Facing the Unknown: People Welcome 51

6. The Universally Human: Great Oneness 57

7. Our Responses to the Elements: Five Pivots 67

8. Further Responses to the Elements: Earth Five Meetings 73

9. Conversations with the Elements: Exchange Pledges 83

10. The Elements under Stress: Not at Ease 91

11. The Line between Balance and Imbalance: Heavenly Pivot 99

12. The Tide of Fate: Dark Gate 105

Afterword: Healing in Death: Soul Door 115

About the Author

Nora Franglen has a degree in Modern Languages from Cambridge University, and worked as a translator whilst bringing up a young family. Her own experience of five element acupuncture led her to study at the College of Traditional Acupuncture, Leamington Spa, UK, and she continued her postgraduate studies there under J.R. Worsley. She was Founder/Principal of the School of Five Element Acupuncture (SOFEA) in London from 1995–2007 and continues her teaching through her practice, through postgraduate work in the UK, Europe and China, and now through her blog, norafranglen.blogspot.com. She lives in London, UK.

INTRODUCTION

The aim of these thoughts is to provide insights into what I have learned from my years of practice as a five element acupuncturist. Each practitioner of sufficient experience will devise the methods by which they work based upon that experience, and there is something in this gathering of experience which cannot be taught directly, but has in some way to be gleaned from our own experiences and from those who have preceded us and have more years' work for us to draw upon. But ultimately we each have some personal input which makes our way of treating peculiarly our own, and this is how it should always be, unless we are to think of ourselves as robots. At some level, if each of us can add something, however small, which is uniquely our own contribution, this moves our discipline forward and enriches it, keeping it a living, breathing discipline.

And so what is that accumulated learning which I bring into my practice room, and which I want to pass on as completely as is possible to whoever wants to listen and learn? At its very heart lies my conviction of what I see as a perception of pattern to the way in which we respond to pressures upon us. Initially, I regarded acupuncture as a purely medical discipline, on a par with other medical systems. I thought that what I was studying was something that would show me how to heal, make whole, what was physically broken, using the instrument of a needle to do this. Looking back now I believe I must have equated what I was doing with what a doctor did, the only difference being in the tools we used and the philosophical framework underpinning what we did. What I now see as this somewhat limited vision has expanded as I have learned to understand that the slight headache with which a patient comes to me leads directly down into the deepest areas of human existence. Instead of contenting myself with trying to find acupuncture points to help the headache I have learnt that my search for these points leads me ever deeper into often challenging areas of existence. Initially this was much to my surprise, forcing me to try to find answers to those perennial questions of who we are, why we are here, what we are here to do and indeed whether such questions can ever be answered at all.

But I do not regard our attempts to cast some light upon such deep matters within the context of acupuncture as too daunting a task, with the proviso always that about some things certainty there can be none. I am convinced, however, of the existence of this expression of pattern in my practice of acupuncture, and I have felt it to be my task to attempt to put into words from the viewpoint of acupuncture how this concept of pattern relates to human health. In particular, my task has been directed at understanding in ever greater depth the prism of the elements which are my tools of trade, however unsatisfactory such an eminently practical, earth-bound expression is when applied to the ephemeral, delicate and poetic nature of the world in which these elements weave their infinite and intricate dances of creation.

These thoughts then represent another facet of what I want to pass on of what I have learned, and can be used by other acupuncturists as another approach to what they do, and by non-acupuncturists as an illustration of a way of looking at the human body and soul which may help clarify some of the mysteries of why we grow ill, in body or soul, in the way we do and what can be done to get us well again.

We live in an age of instant knowledge, with the internet the most visible sign of the speeded-up access to this knowledge. In older, more leisurely times, knowledge was understood to be a gift acquired by graft and dedication, and one which recognized the need for acknowledging the experiences of our elders, welcoming the fact that these elders (and were they not also called our betters!) knew something we younger ones did not, and were prepared to hand this over in a form of discipleship or pupillage. This age-old recognition that the handing down of experience is important has now been replaced by other values, which appear to base themselves upon less easily defined factors. The experience of others no longer appears to be regarded as essential in the acquisition of any skill as does a kind of lauded reliance upon the self-acquisition of such skills. This is the spirit underlying much of modern educational theory.

To study a discipline, therefore, which is built upon a bedrock of knowledge handed down personally from the more to the lesser experienced flies in the face of such theories to the extent that the more experienced, among whom I count myself in the field of five element acupuncture, may often be reluctant to show that they do have more experience than their more junior colleagues. One of the dangers here is that the route of transmission of knowledge in traditions based upon the oral and personal handover of such knowledge becomes blurred by a kind of fake self-consciousness, where those knowing more are hesitant to reveal their superior knowledge in case, they have been warned, this undermines the less experienced. Current educational theory appears to encourage students to make their own discoveries as far as possible unaided (but then how often such theories change, as I have witnessed in my lifetime). Those with more experience are to some extent advised to hide this for fear of fuelling the novice's insecurities. Against such a background, much experience and knowledge must inevitably get lost which it has not been thought appropriate to pass on.

As with my other books, these thoughts form part of what I wish to pass on, a handing over of what I have learnt. They are not prescriptive. I am not saying that this is what others should accept, but it offers my experience as food for others' thoughts and experiences. I am quite happy if what I say is disputed, but I want the debate to take place, and owe it to acupuncture that it does, as often as possible and as deeply as possible, with my and others' ideas to feed it, since challenges are always necessary to stimulate the new.

As acupuncturists, we have to start remembering that the foundation for all that we do, the profound philosophy of life upon which acupuncture is based, is concerned with questions relating to how to live a life well, and that acupuncture is merely (merely!) one of the many, many ways in which we can help this process along, correct it when it has gone awry, and prevent such going awry recurring. We fall into bad habits when we imagine that we are only here to do the first of these, to correct what has gone wrong, for in so doing, preoccupied as we are with that rather miserable pocket of our life which goes by the name of ill-health, we fail to put our work into the context of life as a whole, and thus to look at ways of maintaining health. Here we are undoubtedly encouraged in what I would call our malpractice (in its original sense of the word as meaning wrong practice) by the overwhelmingly medically oriented world we inhabit now, which is so slanted towards probing ill-health, that the search for health occupies very much a secondary, not to say non-existent, role, and is rarely considered as an end in itself. This is a mindset to which we as acupuncturists fall all too easily prey, however much we may think we resist it.

I would like what I write to be, instead, a paean to what this ancient Chinese approach to questions of well-being can teach us here in the 21st century and to the potential for leading a good and healthy life, rather than an exposition of the ways acupuncture has devised to overcome ill-health. And this is not merely physical good health, although that is, of course, important, but health of our soul in its widest, deepest context, a far more difficult thing to maintain and to preserve. Soon after I qualified, I started giving evening classes in five element acupuncture to the lay person, and these to my surprise quickly turned into discussions on the meaning of life and our relationships to nature, the world at large and to one another at the deepest level, rather than concentrating on how acupuncture can help sinusitis or a headache. I remember that after 12 evenings together one of my students, rather hesitantly, asked whether I could show them an acupuncture needle, so far from this very basic tool of my trade had our discussions wandered. Acupuncture, the actual insertion of a needle, was far from our thoughts as we explored together the vast realms of the elements and what they contributed to our understanding of human behaviour.

But until we have worked out for ourselves some context in which to place human strivings, human pains and human joys, we cannot address issues of ill-health and what is needed to correct them with any confidence that we will succeed. It is even appropriate to think that we are approaching things from quite the wrong angle if we start from the viewpoint of ill-health rather than from health when a patient first comes to us, for in what direction do we then try to move their energies if we are not really sure what good health is for that particular person, and what is required to achieve it?

Finally, as a very practical person, it seems to me appropriate to tether what I am writing here in that most practical of all aspects of my practice, the acupuncture point itself.* I have therefore enjoyed myself by assigning a point to each chapter of this book, one whose English name in my tradition echoes something I am trying to convey in the chapter. I am sure that others would have chosen quite different points, but one of the advantages of writing a book is that you can do what you like, so I hope my readers will indulge me in this.

---

* I have Rob Ransome to thank for this suggestion.

CHAPTER 1

CHALLENGES OF A FIVE ELEMENT PRACTICE
Listening Palace

One of the interesting things about running an introductory course on five element acupuncture for acupuncturists practising other disciplines, as I have just done, is that I am able to observe the challenges five element acupuncture presents to those unfamiliar with it. This helps me home in on what I see as the essential elements of my practice, for I have had to distil it increasingly into what I regard as its purest components so as not to overwhelm those unfamiliar with it. This is also a salutary exercise, not just because it helps others, but for myself, because it forces me to look at each aspect afresh.

I suppose that each practitioner has their own list of what challenges them the most in their practice, but underlying them all are some which we appear to have in common. Perhaps heading the list is that fear of not getting our diagnosis right, which must be common to all therapists. In acupuncture, there is something about the need to pick up a needle and do something with it, if not immediately at the start of our encounter with a patient, then after what, in the eyes of some therapies, would be considered to be almost indecent haste, which may appear to make this need for speed more urgent.

But we should stop ourselves here, and compare the long, slow process of making a diagnosis which a psychotherapist will undertake, involving many months, if not years, of work with patients, with our own form of diagnosis of a few hours. As five element acupuncturists, no less than any psychotherapist or counsellor, we are attempting to help the psyche enclosed in that body which our needle will be approaching. I still find it rather strange that I can be expected to be able to condense such deep-searching work into the briefest of time frames like that of our first encounter with our patient. Far better to acknowledge that it always, I repeat always, takes time to get to know a patient at sufficient depth for their elements to show their true natures. Unless we accept this, we will put pressure on ourselves to find too quick a solution through a hurried diagnosis which patients themselves often do not expect us to do. At the head of my personal list of challenges, therefore, is the need for me to resist the desire to speed things up rather than to allow them their own cadence.

Next comes a different need, that of combating complacency. So difficult is any work with people, at whatever level and particularly at the deepest level, that we often greet those patients who are apparently giving us little trouble and are well advanced in their treatment with a kind of relieved light-heartedness and casualness that may lead us to overlook things that we should be addressing. We may be lulled into some sort of almost passive participation, taking for granted things which may not really be as a first glance shows them to be. At intervals then, with our longer-standing patients, we need to check ourselves, and deliberately turn ourselves back into the attitude with which we approached these same patients at the start of their treatment, trying to see them with the fresh eyes we had then. I am often surprised at how much then appears slightly skewed, as though the picture of this particular patient I had built up in my mind no longer fitted how they actually are. In other words, I have assumed things without continuing to test my assumptions against the patient's reality.

I realize that buried within these assumptions lies quite a lot of fear, for I think we are all fearful lest what we would like to believe is a firm diagnosis of what is wrong may shed some of its fixed outline, allowing the unknown to creep in, with all that this implies of the need to reassess our initial diagnosis. It is far cosier to remain cocooned in our belief that with this one patient at least we are working on familiar ground, rather than being forced to contemplate the need for a change of direction in our approach. And this change also brings with it the implication that we may initially, God help us, have been wrong in our diagnosis, and this challenges our confidence in our skills. So the temptation is always there to shut our eyes rather tightly to anything which may shake what should always be our somewhat fragile trust in our initial diagnosis. For all initial diagnoses must have hovering over them a large question-mark, until both patient and practitioner can see the evidence of those powerful changes which a deeply correct diagnosis with properly focused treatment will bring about.

Then there is the question of sheer stamina. It is a long haul, this business of ours, certainly not a quick, pop-an-aspirin-in-the-mouth kind of fix. If done properly, we and our patients are in it together for the long term, and this sense of a long road stretching before us, although at one level satisfying as evidence that we must be doing something right, at another level creates its own pressures. The start of any treatment is always exciting, and, though it may, as I have pointed out above, have its own particular challenges, we seem to be able to gather enough resources within ourselves to keep our adrenalin flowing at the right level. It is when we have passed beyond these initial stages, and have reached some kind of an early plateau, that we slow down to draw breath a little. And this is when a slight irritation may creep in when things don't go quite as we planned, and more is demanded of us than perhaps we had expected. We therefore have to learn to pace ourselves properly so that we do not give so much in the first enthusiastic stages only to find ourselves wilting under the pressures of the next, let alone positively depleted by the time things do not quite pan out as we thought they would even further down the line.

Next comes for me one of the most difficult areas, which is how well I can rein back my own expectations of how far any one patient is able or wishes to change as treatment forces change upon them. For every insertion of a needle is an active stimulus of a patient's energies in a direction other than that which these energies were moving along, presumably sufficiently unhappily as to persuade them initially to seek help. Such changes, though apparently demanded as the patient's presence in the practice room bears witness to, may prove unexpectedly unwelcome to these same patients when they put pressures upon them which they had not foreseen.

Regaining balance or achieving a more balanced state demands of a patient harder work than just passively lying down on a couch and awaiting treatment to do its work. If this treatment is to be successful, it requires not just the temporary changes which a needle can bring about, but a kind of focus of the whole being on accepting this change and consolidating it through actions, which may, and usually, do require shifts in all areas of life. Since all energy is one and the needle, in addressing a specific area of this energy, is at the same time helping all the other areas return to balance, the whole of a person, body and soul, has to adjust to these changing energy patterns, and learn to accommodate the often unexpected, and therefore perhaps threatening, pressures which impel towards change.

In every move forward that we take, there is a point when one foot, as it were, is lifted off the ground, but not yet set down further forward, and where we perch unstably on the other and may overbalance. This is a challenging moment for us all, but some of us accept such challenges with eager anticipation, others with fear, just as some of us could never envisage climbing a mountain which others relish the chance to do. But in its own small way, the impetus towards change which the needle induces in us is each time a kind of push up the rockface of our life. The rock may be sloped gently or steeply, but it always involves some kind of climb, rather than a gentle ambling along the plain. And sometimes what is needed of us as acupuncturists is to push the patient forwards to grasp the rock and take the first steps in the climb towards greater balance ahead.

And this is often as frightening a challenge for the practitioner as it is for the patient. Different practitioners accept this challenge more willingly than do others, who may prefer to remain dawdling with the patient on the plain below for longer. We therefore each have to work out how we view our own approach to this particular challenge, and gear our treatment and the way in which we approach our patients to our own abilities. If we prefer a more hands-off approach, the dawdle for longer on the plain, then we will expect far less of our patients than if we feel treatment is there to stimulate more actively towards change, which represents the push up the rockface kind of approach. It will be obvious from what I write that this is mine. But this can be a risky approach, for it may demand more of the patient at any one time than this patient can cope with, and at times more of myself than I may be able to cope with, and then the particular challenge for me is to ensure that I see the need to hold back. Others might instead need to goad themselves and their patients further forward.

Learning to look at the elements in all their manifestations must be thought of as forming the core of five element practice, but even here there are ways of doing this which become increasingly refined with time and practice. I certainly couldn't see in people before what I can see now, as each year of looking adds something and takes away something else from my vision. I see more clearly what is really there because

I am able to strip away more clearly what is not. It is as though the inner gaze of my senses has sharpened so that it penetrates more deeply beneath those layers we all place upon ourselves as a way of surviving in what can be seen as a confusing world.

One of the first lessons I think all of us have to learn is not to see the interpretation of the sensory signals the elements imprint upon us as easy, and to accept this as a necessary and even welcome fact, for it indicates that we are working in a discipline with depths which we constantly need to plumb. We do not tend to rely on feedback from our senses of sight, hearing and smell as much as we do upon our ability to interpret emotional signals. We somehow like to feel that we do know what joy is, or can accurately recognize fear when it occurs. Our tendency is therefore to pin too much on to this area of our diagnosis just because it appears more familiar territory. The first lesson for all newcomers to the field of emotional diagnosis is to beware the traps it can set us. Familiarity with an emotion does not mean that we place it into its accurate five element category. Indeed, its very familiarity, as for example, if we have had much anger swirling around us in our childhood, may make us shrink from recognizing it in our patients, preferring instead to see it, in its primitive threat to us, as something quite else.

So the next stage in this search for the true emotion is to recognize exactly what each of them evokes for us, and in particular what defensive strategies we may have built up to protect ourselves. Only then can we more accurately learn to guide ourselves through this always tricky emotional terrain. And this is no easy thing to do for those who, as well as feeling they are floundering in the unfamiliar world of sensory signals, now have to accept the need to look inwards within themselves before they can accurately look outwards to interpret the emotional signals others send out.

This, of course, is where five element acupuncture comes close to all forms of psychotherapy, and no psychotherapist would dream of approaching a person in a professional capacity without having first done much guided work upon themselves. But many acupuncturists, often trained in branches of acupuncture where the emotional needs of patients are considered to come a far-distant second to their physical needs, or indeed even fail to be of interest at all, find a similar need for self-discovery alien ground, and will need coaxing to work out ways of venturing on to it.

A further area that has to be learnt is that it may seem as though the elements are adept at hiding themselves, whereas in reality they display themselves all the time, much like peacocks strutting in all their glory. Yet to uninitiated eyes this glory is cloaked in mystery, and does not appear to want to reveal itself at first glance. We do indeed seem to see things through a glass darkly, despite feeling that our sight is clear. The rainbow colours of the elements, there within all colours as they are within white, fuse and fade to a uniform colouring, if our sight is thus dimmed. And the same is true of our other senses. It still surprises me how one of these senses of mine may suddenly appear to gain what in visual terms could be called its second sight, and a fresh smell or sound emerge strongly where before I could perceive no specific distinguishing feature. The act of focusing our senses in this way requires tenacity, and does not come easily to any of us, though some may be fortunate in having a particular sense whose accuracy they learn to depend upon more than they can upon the others.

Here again we see the need for hard work, a kind of relentless, continuous application of ourselves in the direction of interpreting one or other sensory signal. We all of us would like to think that there comes a time, hopefully, we feel, very soon after we finish our training, where the scales will fall spontaneously from our eyes and all will be revealed to us in the stark clarity of the elements' colours, sounds, smells and emotions, as though in some magnificent explosion of understanding. How far this is from the truth only our years of practice will show, when the slight liftings of the veil separating us from the reality of others occur only in fits and starts, and are often followed by a time of sensory darkness where what we think we have perceived recedes from sight again. We move forward here slowly, but given time and that application I have talked about, we do progress, often imperceptibly perceiving more than we did yesterday, and a whole lot more than we did a year ago.

I notice this particularly when looking at patients in the company of less-experienced practitioners, for then, as I point out that this patient is demanding much of me, or that person looks rather yellow, I am suddenly made aware, by the incomprehension on my companions' faces, that I am seeing something they cannot yet see, that, in other words, I have passed through a threshold of sensory understanding they have yet to cross. Though gratifying to think how much I have learnt, it is at the same time disturbing, when watching their expressions of concern at what they regard as their sensory blindness, to wonder what further thresholds I, too, have not yet crossed of which I am as yet unaware.

Of course, like all challenging thoughts, it is also stimulating and exciting to become aware in this way of how much more there is always ahead of us, rather than to dwell with complacency on how much we leave behind already done. Nonetheless, human nature being as it is, the constant casting of doubt upon our own abilities which this kind of practice raises can have a drip-like effect upon our self-confidence if we fail to bolster ourselves against too much self-doubt in some way. We need to build up an appropriate support network to help us through what are often difficult stages in our practice, and find for ourselves places and times where such thoughts can be thrashed out and reduced to their proper proportion as forming necessary stages in any meaningful self-development.

I cannot for myself imagine any more demanding work than that of working with the emotions of others, which is what is implied when we talk of holistic medicine, for the word, if it is to mean anything, must mean a medicine of the whole person, and must include that deep area of our life for which the word emotion is only a pale and partial description. And this brings me to my dislike of using the word medicine in conjunction with acupuncture, implying as it does that all that we do is deal with sick people. This is so far from the truth as to be laughable if it wasn't so sad. For to draw acupuncture into the world of the sick in this way is to deprive it of much of its glory. I am at the moment helping translate some commentaries on the Suwen by Elisabeth Rochat de la Vallée from French into English in my other guise as translator, and what is quite clear from these earliest acupuncture texts is that at heart the only thing they consider worth concentrating upon is the health of the whole being, and regard ill-health, the treatment of the sick which is all that Western medicine thinks of, as only half the story, and probably the least interesting half at that. Of far more concern is how each person remains whole in body and soul.

Any treatment to redress imbalances in this healthy state is not then viewed as an end in itself, but forms part of a greater picture of health, and must never be separated from this greater picture. It is from this perspective that I view my day-to-day work. I therefore like to see it, not as pushing back a tide of ill-health increasingly swamping the world, as this larger picture of health is denied or ignored, but as a gentle encouragement and coaxing back to what we can only hope is that original state of healthy living, or residing in the wholeness of the Dao, as the ancient Chinese would put it, which underlies all that acupuncture does. Unfortunately the Dao, with all that it implies of completeness, of things coming to a point of rest within themselves, is often far from our thoughts as we struggle with the many complex problems our patients present us with. But the fact that it is not always, or perhaps hardly ever, at the forefront of our thoughts, does not absolve us from making efforts to keep it there!

CHAPTER 2

THE IMPRINT OF IMBALANCE

Penetrating Inside

One of the delights that my increasing understanding of acupuncture has yielded is a vision of the human body like some balloon responding to the pressures upon it from within and without rather than the fixed image my study of anatomy has given me. I see its contours changing in a constant state of transformation, expanding and retracting in response to the complex movements imparted to them not only by the inhalations and exhalations of our breath, but by no less powerful mechanisms created by the other functions within the body. Thus this body of ours will retract and shrink into itself with grief or expand with joy or anger, relaying its shrinkages and expansions to our flesh and bones in response to changes in the energy pouring through our meridian network. When faced with some evidence of physical distress, I will immediately try to place this into a wider context in which I visualize its presence as an imprint pressed upon the body by unbalanced energies, and try to work out exactly from which out of all our energies this imbalance stems, where and how it reveals itself and, above all, if possible, why.

I will now trace the route of my own thinking, from the appearance of the patient with this particular symptom to the decision to carry out a specific treatment to help it. Perhaps I need to emphasize here that even as I write this I realize that I am distorting slightly the description of what I do, because my first thought is not how to get rid of the hay-fever, for example. Instead, I am concentrating much more on tracing a bigger picture into which I am trying to fit the hay-fever, leaving the hay-fever itself, and, I hope, its eventual elimination, to take its proper place in due course. By that, I mean that I try not to allow myself to be harried into thinking of the hay-fever as the ultimate cause whose effects I am trying to mitigate, rather than an effect of a larger cause elsewhere. This I see as an imbalance, a distortion, a knock, to the serene and harmonious flow of the energies which together create the proper functioning of all my organs, all my body parts, all my emotions and all my thoughts. I try to place my patient's poor nose and poor irritated eyes, which are responding to the extra force nature exerts upon her breathing as the sap rises in spring, within the larger context.

And here we need to remind ourselves of our acupuncture charts with their vertical lines signifying meridians and their numerous dots signifying points, and remember that this is only a two-dimensional representation of a three-dimensional, not to say four-dimensional being, as we change over time, for it depicts an outline of a body with no indication upon it of its inner soul breathing life into every pore. Each of the lines we see should be thought of as passing through each cell, infusing it with different forms of life, and together forming a dense, interlocking unified whole which is that of us captured in a photo, or, better, in a painting in which the artist has attempted to infuse with his soul his perception of our soul within our body. Thus, to think, as we approach needle to skin, that we are doing little more than a needlewoman does as she stitches a hem on a skirt is to do a serious disservice to the wonder of what we are doing. Far better to see the needle as unlocking a mysterious door to an inner world of awesome depth and wondrous complexity, and retain this image within us each time we devise some plan for the treatment we are preparing for our patient.

Nor must we regard the body as a discrete, finite entity, with edges that are clear-cut, a field of activity bounded by the contours of our flesh, a kind of box within which we fit and out of which bits fall or are propelled only by accidents or surgical intervention (a broken bone, an abscess, an appendix removed, a biopsy taken). I have written elsewhere (see *Keepers of the Soul*) of the concept of the fluidity of our body, of its shimmering, ever-changing surface and its responsiveness to the stimulations upon it of the cosmos outside within which it is embedded and from its internal world within, whose shifting shapes press upon its physical structures as they do upon its emotional landscape. As with all that is alive, we are beings in constant stages of becoming, and whereas the word 'being' can appear to imply that we remain as we are at any moment, we know, as much from modern physics as from ancient Chinese wisdom, that nothing 'is', or rather that the state of being, of 'isness', is superseded at each moment by the next second, minute, day, year of constant transformation.

My finger-nails, for example, grow minute by minute and hour by hour, this growth almost invisible to me until I become aware that they need cutting. The same processes are going on elsewhere on both my outside and inside, reflecting different forms of change. Our skin changes more secretly than do our nails and hair, sloughing itself off cell by cell in a way imperceptible to the eye, as do those processes involved in the renewal of worn-out cells in every organ and part of our body. At the deeper levels within us too, all is in flux; our emotions shift, our behaviour changes, we are happy one minute, sad the next, active today, passive tomorrow. Somehow this process of constant transformation proceeds apace within us without our becoming too aware of it, except when it is interrupted or becomes disturbed in some way. And it is when these interruptions or disturbances grow too marked to ignore that their sufferers turn outside themselves for help to such as me.

My work as acupuncturist can be seen as a continuous attempt to assess the point at which what can be regarded as a normal fluctuation in such processes of transformation tips over into a state which requires some intervention from my needle, when, in other words, a condition becomes what we call pathological. It is very difficult to decide exactly when this happens, and different therapies, and even different cultures, will apply different criteria as to what can be regarded as 'normal', that is, within norms which do not require intervention, and 'abnormal', that is, which lies outside these norms and by tradition or by personal judgement of both sufferer and therapist might be thought to benefit from some intervention from one form of therapy or another. Even if we work on the assumption that it is easy to distinguish the normal from the abnormal, which is far from being the case, it seems obvious that we should make some attempt not merely to try to correct the abnormality in some way, which is what all therapies are trying to do, but to fathom its cause to prevent it happening again, for we are not to know whether it will not immediately recur. And this is where the going gets tough, so tough, indeed, that, at a physical level, which is what Western medicine almost exclusively addresses, the concept of prevention of a re-occurrence is not often within its frames of reference, except in certain rather restricted areas where lifestyle advice appears called for (giving up smoking, not drinking too much alcohol, eating healthily, doing sufficient exercise, for example).

But the idea that diagnosis and treatment should include finding a causal link somewhere along the chain from normal to abnormal, from healthy to unhealthy, is somehow missing in the Western medical context, because the philosophical framework which needs to underpin this is missing, too. The links which might seem to connect cause and effect are simply not there in sufficient strength or at sufficient depth to trace effect from cause in any meaningful way. For us to detect this chain, the parts have got to make a whole somewhere along the line, however disrupted by disease or imbalance this whole may now have become. Where Western medical thought lacks a cohesive philosophy to knit this whole together, its Chinese counterpart has no such problem, for to the Chinese the whole is what matters above all, and the parts embedded in this whole are as microcosm to macrocosm, containing within each of them reflections of that whole. Thus to heal a part means addressing healing to the whole. This is a far cry from the healing of the parts attempted by all those discrete Western medical disciplines in their separate renal, or cardiac or gastroenterology departments.

It is far easier to see things medically from the perspective of the whole, if the philosophical foundation regards that whole as encompassing Man within the biggest whole of all, the Cosmos. In Chinese thought, we form a link between Heaven and Earth, with an unbroken line of communication passing to and fro between all three. Even in Western terms we can see, if we choose to think about it, that the physical heaven above yields us light, warmth and the air we breathe, and the physical earth beneath our feet yields us food, water and shelter, and heaven and earth can thus be seen to pass their energies through us in the light, warmth, food, water or shelter they offer us. Less substantially, at the deeper spiritual level, we can perceive the same connecting links passing through us as we experience the deep feelings of being at one with the cosmos in our contemplation of a sunset, or listen to music or look at a painting or merely revel in the joy of being alive on this earth. All that vast area of our life which receives its benediction from those few to whom creative genius has been vouchsafed, the Tolstoys, the Mozarts, the Picassos, the Rodins, the Shakespeares, is nourished through pathways of energy as essential to my being as are the physical pathways linking each of my physical organs to the next.

Therefore the occurrence of some unease anywhere within this whole, whether it be a headache or a heartache, a physical or an emotional pain in the neck, is understood to send a shiver throughout the whole of us. We know that if we have a slightly infected cut on our finger, our body temperature throughout our system, and not just on the finger, will rise as we try to throw off the infection by raising a fever. Here the whole can be seen to come to the aid of the part that is in distress, evidence that anything that happens on one part of us at whatever level of body and soul is immediately registered by every other part.

This guides my approach to diagnosis and treatment at every stage. I try to keep this picture of my patient as whole before me even when he or she is telling me of the part which is troubled or diseased. It is not easy, even as an acupuncturist for me to do this, for we have all been brought up in a predominantly Western medical culture in which the part is given nearly exclusive priority, all these many different parts of us for which medical specialities have been invented somehow threatening to submerge beneath them that whole from which they come so that finally we may forget that there is even a whole buried somewhere.

As an example of this mentality, I remember my dentist being very surprised when I told him that I had managed to treat a tooth abscess in a patient by diagnosing that there was a blockage of energy passing between the Colon and the Stomach meridians, and by needling points on the side of the nose and below the eye. The abscess drained immediately after needling, 'as though you turned on a tap', my patient said, and the tooth needed no further dental treatment, although my patient had been told that extracting it might be the only dental treatment on offer.

What surprised my dentist was the context into which I had fitted the isolated incident of the abscess. In my diagnosis, the diseased tooth, embedded as a tooth is in the body as a whole, had to be addressed by looking at the whole and not merely by treating or removing the diseased part. Context, therefore, is all. I have to find a place for whatever disease or unease my patient presents me with within the physical and emotional pattern of their life in order to trace this particular hitch in the smooth flow of the energies which together go to create them as healthy human beings. Why, I must ask myself, has this particular stumbling block occurred when it did and where it did? To a world view which sees all things as forming part of a pattern, as did the ancient Chinese mind which first enunciated the precepts upon which acupuncture is based, nothing which impedes the flow of the whole happens arbitrarily. There must be some reason for this disturbance, and this must be traced so that the disturbance it causes can be removed. How successfully and completely I can do this depends on my skill as practitioner in interpreting the signals of distress the body and soul send out through innumerable little messages indicating that the flow of energy is impeded in some way.

I have often said to students that all we do as five element acupuncturists is take energy from where it is excessive and direct it to where it is deficient, convert both the too-much and the too-little into the just-right. And, however simplistic such an approach to what I do might appear, it is fundamentally a true statement. Any illness or state of inner stress is to be regarded as an imbalance in some source of energy somewhere within us. In theory, therefore, all we need do is to correct that imbalance for the illness or stress to go away. In practice, there may be times when the imbalance is too deep-seated, the practitioner not adept enough or the patient too unwilling, for the necessary changes to take place.

CHAPTER 3

THE OTHERNESS
OF OTHERS
Assembly of Ancestors

So here is my patient standing before me as a whole human being, a rounded-out version of the outline in my acupuncture chart. How then do I fit his dense outline into the rather empty template the chart offers, whilst also homing in on places along the chart's energy pathways where some focus of imbalance may have accumulated sufficiently to cause distress? Through what door or doors do I enter the complex, confusing landscape of another human being? And now here at last I come to the five elements, for it is the elements that provide the doors through which all things enter life, and form the entry points through which we approach another human being. I will direct you elsewhere (see *Keepers of the Soul*) for a detailed discussion of my personal understanding of some aspects of the elements, specifically as we recognize their qualities in us, but here I will assume that readers already have some basic understanding with which to read what follows.

There are many ways of adding to our understanding of ourselves and of our fellow human beings. I have been privileged to find my way towards one such profound path of understanding, that which opened up to me when I was introduced to acupuncture and its concepts of the five elements as representing different facets of human behaviour. For here I was given for the first time a very clear confirmation of something I had observed for myself, but much more imprecisely until then. I knew that people were different from each other, reacted differently to each other in ways that usually puzzled them, and appeared to be affronted when faced with this proof that not everybody was like them. But until I encountered the philosophy upon which acupuncture is based, I did not fully appreciate why this was so, or even grasp that this was an unalterable fact about ourselves which, in its positive aspects, leads to the extraordinary variety of human behaviour, and, in its negative aspects, to the extraordinary degrees of intolerance we all, I repeat all, tend to show when confronted with the realities of what I call other people's otherness.

At heart I think we all feel uneasy at the thought that others have as much right to be different from us as we have to be different from them, but we probably don't like to put it to ourselves in quite those terms. Instead, we say things like, 'Isn't so and so odd to act as they do?', or, 'I can't understand why you don't just do so and so', or, 'Why do you get so annoyed at so and so? I just think they're funny.' With this in mind, it is instructive to take some time to observe ourselves, and we may be taken aback at how often we show surprise at the behaviour of others throughout the day.

When we analyze this, we can see that it clearly stems from some cherished belief that we, made up of each individual 'I', hold some personal secret to understanding how things should be viewed which we appear to think is denied others around us, whose behaviour we find incomprehensible and thus in some way reprehensible. Nor must we forget that they, in turn, made up of each 'I' out there, will harbour similar feelings of incomprehension about how we behave. If we are honest with ourselves, it is only in our more enlightened moments, when we are sufficiently at ease with ourselves for us no longer to cast our own long shadows over those that approach us, that we are able to stand back sufficiently from ourselves to see others (and ourselves!) in a truer light.

And such moments are rarer than we may care to believe, since we are always apt to be too kind on ourselves, thinking ourselves to be more tolerant and less judgmental than we in fact ever are.

One of the aims of my work with the elements is to continue to delve deeper into the mysterious worlds of ourselves and of those others out there, and in so doing to feed the shoots of greater tolerance. And with such greater tolerance comes a more balanced approach to the lives we lead in such close proximity one with another. Only a hermit in his cave has no need of strategies for helping him cope with the myriad stresses our daily encounters with our fellow human beings cause us. And I suspect even the hermit has fallen prey in his lifetime to conflicts between his needs and wishes and those of others, which may (who knows?) have been the catalyst for propelling him out into the wilderness in the first place! So even he, too, may find some of what follows instructive.

And it is through my fascination with understanding ever deeper the profound symbolic world represented by the concepts of the five elements as they appear in us that I attempt to grasp some of the mysteries of the human being in health and ill-health, and it is through their prism that I try, with my acupuncture needle, to coax ill-health back to health, to bring balance where formerly imbalance reigned.

What can an understanding of the elements teach us about ourselves that we don't already know? Well, above all, in trying to work out how the elements reveal themselves within us, it makes us look much more closely at ourselves and at our fellow human beings than we will previously have done. I have always been fascinated by human behaviour since my earliest days, but with this fascination there came puzzlement as to why people acted and re-acted as they did. In my pre-acupuncture days, then, I was very prone to thinking this behaviour was odd rather than interesting or instructive. I can still remember, as though that day 30 years ago was merely yesterday, the extraordinary jolt of what I like to feel now was a kind of recognition of some profound truth, when, on my first day at acupuncture college, I learnt about the heart and how the ancient Chinese regarded it, and was told that for some people the heart and its functions, within what I was told was its element, Fire, so shaped their life that it impressed physical and emotional signatures upon them. And I still find it comforting for its sheer appropriateness that my journey into the elements should have started from my own starting-point, my own personal position within the Fire element, which is the circle of Inner Fire, as though a direction to my future life was being pointed out to me even though, then, I had only embarked on my studies out of a vague sense of general interest and with no idea at all that I had found my calling. I also recall being surprised at the time that my fellow students were so sure they were studying in order to practice where I only knew that I was studying in order to learn.

And if we begin to recognize some common distinguishing features which help categorize the behaviour of others in such a way as to make it more comprehensible to us, then one of the main benefits, we will find, is the greater degree of tolerance we begin to show towards facets of this behaviour which before we might have described as odd. With this tolerance comes a greater appreciation of the input others can make to our development, by stimulating us and in so doing often niggling at us with the varying degrees of irritation we feel when forced to deal with what is strange to us, for it requires effort from us to reorientate ourselves around the new and the unfamiliar. What all such encounters do, to varying degrees, though, is throw a stronger light upon some of our accepted views of the world, placing some things in sharper relief, whilst reducing others to a less important role, and thereby changing these views, however slightly. My own journey into the world of the five elements initially jolted

me so abruptly that it felt as if almost overnight I had had
to reposition myself totally with respect to my former ways
of regarding human behaviour, and significant shifts and
similar jolts, though perhaps on a smaller scale, have occurred
constantly since then, as my view of others has been given
different colourings with my increasing familiarity with the
elements.

I like to feel that thereby I have become more tolerant
and less likely to dismiss behaviour which differs from mine,
just as I feel I have at the same time, however gradually and
inadequately, human failings being what they are, grown to
understand better what drives me on and what holds me back.
In becoming kinder to others, my own kindness to myself has
grown, so that, though I am much more aware of my own
motivations, I am not quite so impatient with myself when
I become aware of my shortcomings. I think my knowledge
of the elements and of my guardian element in particular has
helped me understand how often I cannot act any differently,
however much I would like to, because, to use an analogy I
have used before, an eaglet cannot emulate a baby sparrow,
in temperament or body, just as an oak cannot bend and
sway like its fellow willow. And if we look at examples from
nature in this way, we may understand a little better that we
are fighting against a law of nature in asking of ourselves and
of others that we and they should alter patterns of behaviour
which may be as alien to us as would be the predatory lifestyle
of the eagle to the sparrow's gentle scrabbling after grains of
food. And there are eagles and sparrows in human guise, too,
as there are willows and oak trees.

At their deepest level the elements can be seen as life in
its different stages of becoming, and it is my contention (as
it is that of others) that for some reason possibly beyond
our understanding, though we all have the right, if not the
duty, to speculate on this, our characteristics as individuals,
our individualities as unique beings, are somehow so closely

associated with one of the five elements that it casts over us, not so much a shadow, for that has negative overtones, but a patina or wash, colouring us for a lifetime as though dipped at conception into that element. Or, if we want to continue the metaphor of an element being a door, as though we are pushed through a specific elemental doorway into the landscape dominated by that element from which we cannot fully escape throughout our lifetime.

To read further and to follow my thoughts further, you will have to accept this as a given, even if you doubt its truth, for it forms the foundation upon which all five element diagnosis and treatment is built, and is the premise underlying what I write here. So taking as read that we each have a close connection with one element, which I call our guardian element, what does this tell us which can help us build up some method of diagnosing and treating imbalances?

What I am trying to do is to place my patient in the widest context I can find. This does not merely mean the context of their personal life, but where that personal life fits into the wider pattern of things. Recently I was reading about an author who found a childhood book inscribed, as we all used to do, with his name, his address, his country and then, beyond this, the world and the universe. It is interesting that so many of us did this as children, as I remember clearly doing myself. Even then, we must have been aware of the awesome size of the cosmos in which we were embedded and were acknowledging this so simply, an acknowledgement we appear to forget progressively as the demands of life seem so sadly to shrink our horizons down to that tiny space we occupy physically, with the slight extension for our families, friends, workplace and other social gatherings which we allow it. We should be aware at all times, as we were as young children, of this great All within which we are embedded, for such an awareness gives our thoughts quite a different dimension, adding relevance and significance and removing pettiness and insignificance. It is a difficult place to reside in, this vast space around and within us, but if we dare to allow ourselves thus to keep our eyes open, we will find we are accompanied into this space by the comforting presence of all great artists, for this is the space they continually inhabit.

I have been immersing myself in Shakespeare this year, determined before I die to have read all his plays and seen them performed, and such is the teeming life he takes me to look at that, when I emerge, the sheer littleness of some of the things I occupy my daily life with astounds me. I feel my world is thereby set more to rights, I am re-aligned, as it were, with what is essential, significant, worthwhile. And though this realignment may not last as long as I would like it to, it nonetheless affects a shift in my perceptions which is of longer-lasting value. And that is how I see the purpose of great art, to make us see things afresh, remove the trivial and keep the essential before us.

In its specifically focused way, perhaps surprisingly to some of us, as it certainly was to me at first, treatment can do this too, for in its alignment of us with all the energies that flow through the cosmos and through us it reinforces our connection with everything around us, and thus, if properly accepted as doing this by both practitioner and patient, extends an awareness beyond ourselves by placing us into a closer relationship with all things. In so doing it gives us a truer perspective from which to view things. When treatment brings about greater balance, then, our view of 'life, the universe and everything' gains greater balance.

I always tell my new patients that when we first come for treatment our energies are slightly (or greatly!) out of kilter, and thus slanted to one side or another, as though symbolically we are walking through life with our heads at an angle. We thus see all things through some kind of distortion, much as we would if we could no longer stand upright and had to lean to one side or another. But our imbalances mean that we are rarely aware that our view on life is tilted to an angle. Instead, on the principle of that wise, old adage of 'All the world is strange, save thou and me, and even thou art a little strange', we instead tend to judge others as being the ones to view things from the wrong angle. It is little wonder, then, that the more out of balance we become, the more we misrepresent the world to ourselves and the less flexibility and insight we have to adjust ourselves to its vagaries.

With good treatment comes this realignment of our energies in relation to what is going on inside us and to what flows towards us from outside. Little by little, we hope, we stand a little more upright, and each shift in our energy brings about a slight shift in the perspective we bear on things. Those strange people out there, whose oddness we were amazed at, now take on an increasingly less strange appearance as our assessment of their behaviour changes its angle. When we regain balance as far as any human being can, we may well begin to see that it is we who slanted our relationships, our opinions, our behaviour, more than we were aware we were doing. The more upright we stand, with our energies flowing in the channels they should and with the strength they should, the more upright is our perception of what is going on around us, and inevitably the more tolerant we begin to be as we start to accept all the complexities of our engagement with the world around. The more out of balance we are, the more starkly black and white we see everything as. The more complex shadings of grey come only with greater insight.

CHAPTER 4

DOORWAYS TO THE ELEMENTS
Spirit Path

We now need to step back a little, whilst keeping before us in our mind's eye a picture of a person as a whole, the person coming for treatment for the first time. To me she is a kind of blank canvas very similar to that which faces a painter attempting to draw her portrait. At first I can see nothing but a kind of emptiness, a void, until my vision gets sharper, and then slowly I begin to paint in physical and emotional expressions so that after a little time I think I will be able to describe some salient physical or emotional features, however sketchily to start with. Something is emerging from the canvas, as though a picture is starting to draw itself. I may be able to add touches here and there, and with time, and it always takes a great deal of time and patience, I contribute to the drawing by focusing my questioning and 'drawing out' from my patient aspects of herself which she allows herself to show me once we have developed sufficient trust with one another.

And now I need to turn to what I have learned so far to help us move to the next step. For this particular patient, though unique in her attributes, yet has features and characteristics which are common to all mankind, and these are captured for me as an acupuncturist in symbolic form in the acupuncture charts which hang on my clinic walls. So as my patient describes to me something of her life, and something of the physical pains and emotional stresses she suffers from, my mental eye superimposes upon what she is telling me that picture of energy lines flowing through and round her (and also, we know, deep within her). As she describes a particular area of physical or emotional pain, my mind tries immediately to make some link between what she is telling me and those lines. Sometimes this link is immediately very strong, sometimes it is so weak or non-existent that I can see little or no connection between the disturbed energies she is describing to me and the template of energy lines I am attempting to fit these to. But if I can detect some pattern at work here, I am taking my first steps towards making a diagnosis on which to base my treatment plan.

In the example of the tooth abscess I discussed with my dentist, in addition to pinpointing the meridian and the site of the acupuncture points along that meridian where the abscess appeared to have burst out, I noted the following: the patient complained of nausea, his colouring was whiter than usual and his immediate superior was giving him a difficult time at work. If I relate each of these signs of distress to my knowledge of the pathways of energy shown pictorially on the chart, each told me something which I then had to draw together into some meaningful context. From all these signs I recognized that both his Metal and Earth elements showed some distress (bloated stomach, excessively white colour, emotion of grief towards his colleague's lack of respect for him). That these two elements were involved in the imbalance was corroborated by what my pulse reading had already made me aware of, which was an inequality in the energy flow between two of the officials, Colon and Stomach, at the superficial level of the body, the Wei level, indicating that the end of the Colon meridian was blocking energy which should be flowing towards the Stomach meridian. Taken altogether, this led to a damming up of energy around the nose and cheek, the physical expression of distress at both physical and emotional level. This called for the points at the end of the Colon, beside the nose, and at the start of the Stomach, below the eye, to be needled to re-establish a good energy connection between the two officials and the elements they represent within us. The treatment was completed by putting the patient back in control using some foundation points on his guardian element, which happened to be Wood.

Afterwards, on reviewing all the facts and with the outcome of treatment confirming my diagnosis, I could see that the abscess had formed because of this blockage of energy, creating a focus for the accumulation of what we call harmful energy, in the form of pus, and with it causing great pain. The path leading from the accumulation of blocked energy to the formation of the abscess is fairly easy to trace, and the treatment at one level is simple. The picture becomes more complex if we delve further, and enquire why such a blockage might have occurred in the first place. It is not enough just to say that it did, as a dentist might. At the deeper level, the distress shown by the Metal element causing the blockage to the Earth element would appear to provide a more satisfactory answer. Could it be that the affront to the patient's feeling of self-worth, as represented by a weakening of the Metal element and its officials, might lie at the heart of this imbalance, and be expressing itself through the abscess as though through the release of some safety valve?

If so, merely treating the abscess by relieving the blocked energy will only provide temporary relief. To prevent the same thing recurring, I need to check how deeply ingrained in our patient is the fear of ridicule he suffered from so strongly at the time of the first infection. I released the physical accumulation of pent-up aggression as expressed by the abscess by needling the points which I did, but I may have to deal with a deeper feeling of pent-up emotional energy through further treatment to ensure that my patient regains the feeling of self-worth formerly lacking in him. This I will do by ensuring that his guardian element, Wood, is boosted by focused treatment which props him up from inside, and helps him guard against feelings of self-doubt. One way of doing this is also to help him see how far he was affected by the troubles at work, and discuss with him ways in which he can avoid the kind of emotional attack his Metal element experienced and which eventually led to the abscess. I will therefore always have to keep a close look-out to ensure that his Metal element remains sufficiently strong not to weaken in the future.

In this patient the doorway to helping his Metal element will be that of Wood. In quite another person, whose guardian element may be Fire or Water, the same blocked energy, and therefore a similar abscess, might have developed, but its root cause may stem from imbalances in the Fire or Water elements rather than in Wood.

These lines and dots on the chart represent something very profound to me, something which has underpinned all that I do, so that now I no longer see the chart as I did when I started my studies, as something representing a physical body, much as a Western anatomy or physiology chart represents that body, but as being so much more than the mere body that I almost forget that it is the body which I needle. This is because my concept of the elements and of their messengers, the 12 officials, with their meridian pathways like some postal system passing relays of messages to and fro, has widened so much as to make it impossible now for me to think back to a time when the chart did not represent that density of thought and concept which helps me now approach the profound complexity of the energies which feed us all.

This act of translating the symbolic representation of a human being in my chart into the realities represented by each of my patients has become increasingly automatic to me that, to examine it, I have to unravel my thought processes, as I did for my patient with a tooth abscess, to help me unpick stage by stage the processes which help me eventually decide upon a schema for treatment. In the few minutes between a patient's appearing in my clinic and my selection of his/her treatment, what I am doing is trying to fuse together what I already know about my patient from previous treatments and what I am now being told about them, both in their words to me and in the information my senses are gathering for me. The next step in the process I go through to select a treatment is to set this against the template of the chart I keep in my head.

It is a hard task to round out our patients in this profound way in the comparatively brief time we are given with them in the practice room, nor can we expect that our ability to do this comes at our first encounter with them, or indeed even at our fifth encounter. We need to work on a time scale much longer than that which we might give treatments of a purely physical nature, and think rather of giving ourselves the kind of time traditionally granted psychotherapists and their patients, and accepted as being necessary to gain insights into the depths of a person's psyche. For we need this time to gain the understanding our patients want of us, and to help our acupuncture skills match what is asked of us.

We can see each visit of our patients as forming part of a never-ending process of diagnosis to which the patient brings that new person with his/her new experiences and the changes such experiences have wrought upon them since the last visit. Some of these new experiences and new changes will, I hope, be the result of treatments they have received from me. Others will be those that life outside confronts them with, and which in turn have to be assimilated and dealt with by my patient and incorporated into my thinking about how to select the treatment I will give. We should never think that our diagnosis is definitive, final or unalterable, for that implies something static, whereas the person we are trying to help is constantly changing and transforming. This change and transformation changes and transforms the diagnosis and thus the treatment called for.

In every diagnosis, too, we have to be careful that, once having decided on the doorway we have learnt to label as the Wood, Fire, Earth, Metal or Water element through which we will choose to enter the domain particular to that patient, we do not then lock it firmly behind our patient, as though what lies behind is no longer of interest to us. For if we really look closely at each of the limitless number of past, present and future people we meet, we know quite well that, although they will have some very general characteristics in common with others of the same element, which we learn to describe in basically imprecise terms such as the colour yellow or the emotion grief or a shouting tone of voice, in each person the yellow colour or expression of grief or shouting voice is totally unlike any others'. And this is because it is as unique an expression of that particular unique person as is his or her genetic make-up. Into this yellow, grief or shout is poured an admixture of qualities utterly specific to that person, although these characteristics will have some features in common which help us distinguish the dominant elemental sphere which is stamping its signature upon them.

How often, too, we find ourselves taken aback by some hitherto hidden quality in a person which we may have previously thought indicated one element, only to discover on closer acquaintance that tiny facets of what we had taken to be pointers to the Wood element are instead indications of the presence of the Metal element, a sharpness, for example, now allocated its true origins as emerging from Metal's acute need to get the true value of things right, rather than Wood's equally acute need to print structure upon its understanding of the world. For it takes time to get to see our patients as they truly are, and it is good to see the process of treating as a way of getting to know another person, of forming a better acquaintance with them, akin to creating the seeds of a long friendship with the elements within that patient. Only with time will we, and the elements within us, relax sufficiently to allow ourselves to see our patients clearly, and only with time will they, and the elements within them, relax sufficiently to reveal their true natures, much as we need time to deepen any relationship.

CHAPTER 5

FACING THE UNKNOWN
People Welcome

When we are faced with the need to open up to another human being about ourselves, whether this be initially merely about some physical pain or even, somewhat more riskily to start with, about some deeper unease, we move into what might well seem to us to be dangerous territory, for we do not know how the listener will respond to what we are telling them. Unfortunately all too frequently many of us have experienced some kind of inappropriate response to something we have told somebody else, either as part of a professional encounter or in our personal lives. This kind of response will range from the 'How terrible, but cheer up, things can only get better' variety, to more subtle ways of denying us the right to feel as we do, of the 'I can't understand why you don't just...' kind of response. These indicate all too clearly to us that the listener chooses not to venture into our terrain of experience or only wishes to see things from their own personal perspective.

All such comments effectively close the door on our divulging more. In a more professional, rather than purely personal, situation such as those I have described above, they will probably be more subtly expressed but have the same effect of silencing us and making us feel we are rather odd to feel as we do. It takes great skill for the listener to stand, as it were, outside themselves and work out ways of moving into the speaker's space. Having all of us, I am sure, had just such unhappy experiences of denial of our right to express how we really feel, the first encounter with a practitioner, and often quite a few further encounters, will initially be viewed with much trepidation, for our patients may well be asking themselves if we, too, will be unable to hear them.

If we are being honest with ourselves, those first interactions with a new patient are always quite frightening for us, too, for none of us, even the most experienced practitioner, feels comfortable with uncertainty, and a new patient is an unknown, uncertain quantity. It requires courage to tackle such uncertainties head-on again and again in our practice, and perhaps more courage than we are aware of. This may be one of the reasons why practitioners may fall by the wayside altogether, or retreat into stock responses to emotional demands upon them behind which they feel they can safely shelter, without allowing too many demands to be made upon their capacity to place themselves outside their own particular emotional sphere and venture into unfamiliar areas, with all the challenges this involves.

Indeed, it could be argued that the whole area of work which entails our deliberately working within the boundaries of another's personal space, as any form of therapy which reaches within the world of psychotherapy does, is fraught with risk, to both the patient and the practitioner, risks rarely acknowledged because their implications can be thought to be too threatening. If, as I believe strongly, the realms in which another person acts out their life should be regarded by them and us as sacred space, then to work within all the many different sacred spaces into which each new patient invites us requires some deep adjustment to the way in which we approach others in our everyday roles. In all the different kinds of training available for work in the fields of these therapies, much play is made of the need for boundaries and for respect for the patient/client, and many structures are put in place to render these awesome, often wild and untameable places where reside other human beings tamer and less fearsome, by elaborating procedures which ease entry. We have formulae for charging our patients, for making appointments, for cancelling appointments, but behind these lies the unknown terrain on which we have been asked by our patient to set foot, and it is not idle to see this exploration with the patient somewhat in the nature of that famous picture of the first landing on the moon. For here, too, the therapist alights in completely unknown territory.

We do much better in our work if we acknowledge all this to be so, rather than denying it, as there is a temptation for us all to do, for do we not all like to consider ourselves to be civilized, balanced human beings who should not be affrighted by the areas in which we work? Many, though, are the approaches to what we, as therapists of any kind of discipline, do, and these range from our viewing work as a straightforward transaction in which we offer a known something which the patient accepts, or does not, and which helps, or does not help, the patient, to the other end of the scale, where I like to think I position myself, where what I seek to offer is far from straightforward, and has to be worked hard for, and what the patient receives from my work is sufficiently complex to be constantly challenging. For touching the depths, in both patient and practitioner, is a far from comfortable experience, and I often ask myself, even now after so many years, why I put myself so on the rack each time I enter the practice room. Of course, I usually give myself the same answer, 'Because the rewards of helping another to greater balance, that of realigning them with the true course of their own life, have become so essential a part of my life, giving it a value far beyond its often meagre financial rewards, that I can no more think of stopping working, of "retiring", as many of my friends have already done, than I can of stopping breathing or feeling.'

For I feel called to do what I do, as others are to other areas of human experience. It is my calling. And how do I define a calling? Perhaps it is easier to think first of what it is not. It is not merely a job of work, something we do to earn money to survive. It is more than that, for in the very word itself is buried a hint of some power outside ourselves which summons us. I found myself almost writing the words summons us to arms, because I experience that summoning as containing within it challenges I have to confront and battles I have to win. To have a calling is not a comfortable thing to have, nor does one rest in a comfortable place to fulfil it. Far from it. Indeed, I experience it often as a form of curse, and a burden I would sometimes like to shake off, so heavy can be its responsibilities. For if we are not to deny it, we have to be true to it, and the path to its truths lies often over very stony ground, with many a hidden danger lurking to trip us up. We have to win by hard work the right to deem ourselves true to whatever calling we feel we have been drawn to.

A calling is often also described as being a vocation, and yet this word has become debased by too frequent and too inaccurate use, as the most serious words often are, because I suspect their overuse, like any overuse, reduces their sharp and often uncomfortable edges. And thus we have all those training courses coming under the heading of vocational training which are merely different ways of helping people acquire all sorts of technical skills. Nothing here can resonate with that deeper meaning of being called to do something, although it may well be true that the word can be applied to those, of whatever profession, for whom that profession represents a summons, be that a summons to become a plumber or a summons to become a solicitor. And yet there are, I suspect, different gradations of calling, passing from the desire to acquire and exercise a skill and moving to a somewhat different level where the fulfilment of a desire to do something answers to some deeper imperative.

This is the kind of calling whose summons I have heard and responded to, and in that deeper imperative, I have found, lies hidden much heartache, for unlike the plumber or the solicitor, although here I may be misconstruing their approach to their work, there is something I am called upon to do which lies beyond or beneath or above the actual exercise of the skills I have acquired. My calling makes me restless and leaves me no peace, no time when I can lay it aside and forget about it, for it itches constantly at me, making demands that accompany me throughout all that I do. Since my particular calling as five element acupuncturist bears within it its own interpretation of the different manifestations of human behaviour, at each encounter with others, in the bus, in the street, at a party, some pull is exerted by it which tugs me to another level, and the everyday person disappears, however briefly, within a wider, more all-encompassing being which is me exercising my calling. And it takes some effort on my part to disengage myself again, as that higher imperative lays its demands upon me.

CHAPTER 6

THE UNIVERSALLY HUMAN
Great Oneness

It appears to be a human longing to want clear boundaries and parameters for what we do, and, if we are not careful, this need can extend to what we do in our practice. In our yearning for certainties, we want our patients, too, to have fixed boundaries, and lock them within these by phrases such as, 'he is a passive-aggressive person', or, in a five element acupuncture context, 'her element is Wood', without in our minds mentally adding some necessary modifier to characterize the unique qualities which this particular person represents. There are many, many passive-aggressive people, whose passivity and aggression have a nature all their own, as there are many, many different Wood people whose Wood-like qualities have their own unique imprint. It is clear that we need large labels of some kind into which we fit some of our learning, certainly at the start, but with ever-widening experience these labels, too, widen, stretching themselves and changing their shape to fit the unique shapes of the people they are trying to encompass.

It requires great flexibility on our part to allow such elasticity to the categories within which we need initially to place people, in whatever discipline we work, and we may be tempted as many are, and as I often am, to hold too rigidly to the simple, and therefore rather crude, templates we first start with, because flexibility demands too much of us, leading us, once again, into those unsafer areas in which lurks the unknown. To say that Wood's emotion is anger, and immediately to categorize all who show anger as belonging to the domain of Wood, may appear safer than to try to work out which kind of anger a person is showing, with all that this brings with it of continuing uncertainty. Is it a fiery type of anger or a cutting type? Does it explode outwards towards others or inwards towards the person expressing the anger? Is it therefore more of an anger coming from another element perhaps? All these aspects of this particular expression of anger need to be looked at carefully, but if we do not feel we can answer these questions easily, and thus have to remain a little while longer in the realms of the unknown, we may find such continuing uncertainty disturbing. We may then feel it to be safer to enclose our patient's anger tightly within a Wood box and turn quickly away, lest something new and unexpected rattles our decision.

If the patient then does not improve with this diagnosis, we may be tempted to dismiss the queries this raises with statements such as 'the patient doesn't want to change', or 'whatever I do doesn't seem to help the patient', for fear that in amending our first diagnosis we are opening a Pandora's box. For a Pandora's box is indeed what each of us is to another person, an unknown out of which may pour the unexpected, the challenging or the downright chilling. All of these may form part of what our patients gradually show us as they allow us to come to know them. And none of this must shock or disturb us, however shocking or disturbing what is revealed to us may appear to be. For, to no-one is the dictum, 'there, but for the grace of God, go I', more pertinent than to me as an acupuncturist, who has been given the task of seeing what can be regarded as universally human in each human being who comes to me for help.

The universally human is what underlies all of us, and makes possible our communications one with another, for without this common core we would be too alien to each other to understand what the next man is trying to tell us.

Some common links stretch across the divide between one human being and another, even those most distanced from one another. In this respect, I always find it reassuring when I watch those TV programmes on encounters with remote tribes in the remotest regions on earth, and find how striking is their resemblance to me, sitting here in the heart of a large metropolis, as they laugh with glee at the same jokes, and show the same care, love and hate for each other that I show. Perhaps the ways in which such expressions of love, care and hate are shown may differ somewhat, as no doubt they do between me in London and those as close as Paris, but their essential nature remains the same as to be totally familiar expressions for me watching them many thousands of physical miles away and perhaps many thousands of years' difference in terms of whatever stage of development we may like to think our 'civilized', urbanized society has reached.

It is this deep, underlying common core within all humanity which calls out for healing when we grow sick, rather than the superficial, the socially moulded part of us. And this core is formed of the interlocking, intertwining, intercommunicating of those basic components, the five elements, as expressions of the whole, the Dao, within us. Viewed in this way, as we must, if we are to help another human being to rediscover and maintain his/her wholeness, the elements must be regarded in the widest, deepest way possible as putting us in touch with what is universal within us, at the same time as revealing what is essentially totally individual, a paradox if ever there is one, and one which has been puzzling me ever since I started regarding the uniqueness of each of us as an expression of the unique interactions of the elements within us.

We are not clones of each other, our very genetic make-up so individual that it distinguishes us one from another so clearly. And yet there are human genes which we have in common, as there are their equivalents, elemental imprints, which we all carry with us in the structures of our bones, flesh and organs. Beyond this, lying in layers, as it were, above this common pool of our elemental inheritance, is what makes us unique, in the shape of slightly different expressions of our common core. My laugh is like no other's, but when I and another laugh it is recognizable as laughter by anybody listening to us, and yet... My fear and my companion's fear as we are both stopped at the airport for a scan are recognizably what another would call fear, and yet... And it is in this 'and yet...', this difference in quality, where we as acupuncturists have to work. What, within the common, is specific to that one patient of mine? What, under my laughter or my fear, differs from my neighbour's? And, then, how do tracing these differences to some differing qualities within the properties of the elements within us help me to help my patients?

The differences are ascribed, in element terms, to very specific qualities with which the elements within us endow us as gifts (or curses!) at birth and in early life, and which then, as we grow, imprint upon us ever more emphasized distinguishing marks, until eventually they form the mature human being, capable, we hope, of bringing these blessings to their full potential in creating a worthwhile life. And capable, too, we hope, of confronting any curses which may have accompanied us into life, in the shape of those facets of our inheritance which may appear to dog us and pull us down. I am thinking here of a home life already disturbed before we arrive, or inherited health problems or problems which our early nurturing may imprint upon us and which hinder our well-being and happiness. All these hurdles are there to be overcome and for us to deal successfully with as part of our development, and either add to our growth or to our diminution if we fail to confront them.

And here the strength of our elemental structures comes to our aid, and with it the adjustments that acupuncture can bring to the elements' balance within us. What, then, are the particular areas of life over which each element extends its influence in this way?

The categories of the elements cannot unfortunately be regarded simply as neat little boxes with clear outlines, delineated one from another, with one green, the next blue, as it were, and thus each with defined qualities. At their edges they meld into one another, much like colours of the rainbow do, so that, though when seen from afar there is an appearance of blue or green, on closer inspection these distinct colours start to fuse together, moving imperceptibly from one band to the next. In much the same way, an element, though in some vital respects sufficiently distinct in characteristics as to be distinguishable from the next, loses its defining edges as it merges into the next or is impinged upon by another element, plunging us often into despair when we cannot differentiate something which might initially appear so obvious as grief from joy, or a sad tone of voice from an angry one. If you shut your eyes slightly, and look at things through half-closed eyes, what you first saw takes on quite a different aspect. Thus grief may be parading as hysterical laughter, a white colour be masked by a yellow, one smell be camouflaged by another. In this fluid world of ever-changing shapes which separates the melting outlines of our energies as life presses against us and we press against life, nothing can be positively stated as being so and not something else. It is usually so and something else.

And yet, beneath these fluid forms there exists something stable, for we are, after all, ourselves and no other, and our bodies and our souls have characteristics which are ours and not those of anyone else. But this something that is us is nowhere near as fixed as we would like to think it is, and we must allow it its fluid outlines if we are to be true to the nature of our being. To attempt, then, to imprison the shifting nature of our energies within the static, fixed confines of words, as I am trying to do here, is thus somewhat to falsify them. What is needed is an imagination which removes the stark edges of the words with which I am describing the elements, and replaces them with something more mobile which can expand, contract and change shape to reflect the image of a body's energies with its moving outlines, as though these words and these pages are immersed in water so that their edges dissolve, fade and meld into one another. It requires an approach all its own if we are to work easily within such an often blurred environment, whose apparently fixed edges shift even as we look at them. It is thus that we need to regard the elements, as shifting, moving spaces, which differ from one another but absorb differing qualities from one another so that finally they create the unique human being that is me at this moment, but shift again to create me in the next moment of my existence.

And because we are all movement, an infinite number of physical cells fusing together to create our physical and emotional structures in a jostling pattern, resembling those pictures of magnified cell structures seething with life which we see in science programmes on TV, the slightest knock shifts the structures of the whole of our being and the slightest re-adjustment, in our case with the needle, can shift these same structures back into a more balanced shape. Each insertion of the needle, under the command of the acupuncturist, is an attempt at some form of ordered realignment of energy. The order is imposed by the elements as they exercise control over the areas of our being over which they rule. We have seen that they are five aspects, five expressions, of the whole which is each of us, and where we detect disturbance within a particular area of control that is where we direct the work of readjustment through our needles. It is because of the lack of absolutely clear differentiation between the different areas of control which I have discussed above that our decision as to which point of entry into the domain of the elements to choose is initially so difficult to make, and must always be tentative to start with. In effect, by focusing our treatment upon one element, it is as though we send out a question to the band of elements out there in that patient of ours, asking them whether or not this element is their master, and then we sit back to await their reply.

So how do I start to recognize that I have entered, for example Wood's domain? Of the many indicators, two stand out. The first are the sensory and emotional signposts laid down for us over the centuries to help orientate ourselves in this complex and often confusing landscape, the colours, sounds, smells and emotional signatures which the elements imprint upon us through the work of their officials within us. Thus the Liver and Gall Bladder send their imprints to every cell, as we know when they are sick and we become jaundiced, and our bodies take on a yellowish-green colouring. To acupuncturists, too, such imbalances will also be emotionally visible, as everyday language recognizes when they describe somebody as feeling jaundiced in spirit. Such signatures, when unhealthy as in jaundice, point us towards a Wood element in trouble, or, when healthy, towards one that is flourishing.

A second important indicator is found in the change treatment effects if I am directing it correctly at the Wood element, and its officials respond clearly by showing some alteration, some move towards greater balance. Such changes can be both subtle or clearly obvious, a slight shift in emotional temperature, a softening of hardness, or an abrupt decision to change the direction of a life by giving in notice at work or deciding to take a holiday. The degree of each of these shifts is irrelevant, providing that, together, they contribute to a move towards balance, and here the sensory indicators will also add their bit, revealing a similar move towards greater harmony.

There are other indicators, too, which depend upon interpreting change, but this time not in the patient, but in ourselves as we respond to the person before us. We have to look at the way in which the presence of this person changes how we are in terms of the reactions which the appearance of another human being always arouses in us, and, in the case of a patient after treatment, we need to look at whether such changes show that the element being treated is in a healthier state. And what kind of a reaction do they stimulate? The flickering energy field in all of us not only causes a jostling amongst all those tiny components of our own being that make us who we are, but extends outside us, too, like some form of radiation, meeting and imprinting itself upon those around us. The nature of this imprint of another upon us, and inevitably, too, of us upon that other person we are relating to, forms a crucial part of our interpretation of the balance of the elements within both the person and ourselves. And learning how to allocate our reactions correctly to the sphere of one element or another provides another signpost on the field of the elements which it will be helpful for us to follow.

This raises a further question which is where we position ourselves in relation to the elements within us as practitioners. We cannot ignore the force which our own energies will exert, nor deny that this can distort our perceptions of what is really going on in the patient. That is why it is so important to make correct distinctions between what we ourselves bring to the encounter and what the patient brings. We are, after all, not here as practitioners to focus upon our own needs, but must remain aware that these, too, have to be accounted for. It is useful to ask ourselves such searching questions as, 'Do I enjoy the power my work potentially gives me?', or 'Do I always shy away from close contact with patients who make me feel inadequate?', for in our willingness to address such often awkward issues lies our ability to concentrate upon our patient's needs. All encounters with patients trigger personal reactions within us, and learning to distinguish our balanced from our unbalanced responses forms a fundamental part of the skills we need to develop. When our response is balanced, it can teach us a lot about our patients, and through them the elements; when unbalanced, it can only teach us something more about ourselves, hardly what our patients are paying us to do!

CHAPTER 7

Our Responses to the Elements

Five Pivots

With all this in mind, it is now time to look at the elements from the perspective of how I feel in myself when a dominant element in another person exerts pressure upon me, showing how this has helped me to define a little more for myself some of the qualities that element brings to its encounters. The Wood element is a good starting-point, because it has such a very clearly-defined, 'in your face' kind of energy, and certainly does not shrink from its encounters with others, as some other elements do. It is with this element that the yang, outgoing energies start their rise in nature in spring, and it brings to its encounters a quality of upthrust, making its effect upon us direct and immediate, and thus evoking an equally direct and immediate response from us in return. These responses will vary in as many ways as there are people engaging in such encounters, but they fall into a few main categories, ranging, at one end of the spectrum, from some kind of avoidance of such direct contact, expressed as a desire to get out of the way, right through to its opposite, a desire to push back, by means of a counter-thrust. In between these, there lies a range of more muted responses.

Where each of us positions ourselves along this scale of responses will depend upon many factors involved in our own make-up, but it is important to know where we fit on this scale, so that we can assess which of our own personal issues we bring to the encounter. We can never set ourselves aside, nor should we, as our reactions and impressions form an essential part of any diagnosis, but we must look to see how far our reactions are due to what we bring to the encounter and how far they are due to what the patient brings, before we can interpret the patient's responses correctly to help our work. We have to learn to recognize what a balanced reaction within us is, and here, in the case of Wood, to help our learning we can do no better than observe closely our responses to the advent of spring. For some, the burgeoning buds provide relief as a sign of the end of winter, for others they represent the advent of new life for which they may feel ill-prepared. If we translate this into the same energy expressed this time not by a bud in nature but by a bud in a human being, which is another way of describing Wood's action within us, then both the feelings of welcome relief and of threat are possible reactions we may feel. We could symbolically translate our welcome to spring in human terms as a happy engagement with the other person's Wood energy, a brisk to-and-fro, or a tit-for-tat passage of energy between us, more in the nature of a kind of healthy jousting. On the other hand, we may translate the threat we feel as an advance warning that we need to evade something, inducing a backing away, an instinctive desire to avoid just that head-to-head encounter the welcoming group revelled in. We learn gradually from experience to work out our own template within which to fit our emotional responses, and make our own assessment of whether such and such a response slots into what we can call our Wood template or not.

I therefore set out below my own such template as a kind of guide, but must leave readers to decide from their own experience of observing their reactions how far this is appropriate, if at all, to their responses. If nothing else, it will help pinpoint the kind of sifting process which has to go on within us as we deal with an encounter with another, and we pass it through our own personal assessment grid as though through a sieve. What we are looking for then is not, as with sieved flour, what has fallen through the sieve, but the residue which remains behind, those remnants relating to our particular take on an element which represent that element's effect upon us. It is as though our sieve has an adjustable mesh which we change as we try to assess each element.

Now let us take a look at the distinguishing features of my Wood template which help me work out how far what I am experiencing relates to the Wood element rather than to any other element. The first thing I notice is likely to be the feeling I described as though something is pushing against me. I experience an impact, followed by a slight recoil as I try to regain balance, and then I feel a need to push back. I can feel, too, something within me tighten, my jaw and my hands clench a little in response, as though I am preparing, however briefly, to attack. All this indicates to me that some action appears to be demanded of me, making it impossible for me to remain passive in the face of this. If we look at the range of responses, it would appear that I take up a position at the point of the spectrum of reactions which responds by wanting to stand my ground. The moment I become aware of this response it raises a slightly disturbing feeling in me, that of being in some contest I don't want to get involved in, and I try to disengage quickly. I find I do this sometimes by shifting eye contact, by a word intended to defuse something I feel going on between us, or, as I learn to pinpoint my responses more accurately, by giving a kind of little inner smile as I become aware of what is happening and gain some pleasure in knowing where my reaction is coming from.

There are many physical echoes, too, in different parts of my body. I feel my eyes engaged directly, for in such an encounter I am usually being looked straight in the eye, pinned down, as it were. I have already noted that my hands have clenched slightly. My body is as though on alert, having experienced a push that has moved it slightly backwards, and it now tries to regain its balance with a counter-push. And the word 'counter' occurs frequently in my description of my reactions, indicating a need for some kind of counter-weight to offset the weight I feel pressing upon me. I may also capture evidence of some quickness of movement in my Wood sieve, again indicating an energetic thrust forward. We have seen it already in the feeling I have of being pushed. Here this extends to the space around a person, for movement can be described as a way we have of pushing the space we occupy aside to allow our passage forward.

There are many different ways of moving, different speeds, different positions of the body as we move, all revealing something. We can move sinuously, abruptly, quietly, slowly, quickly or with small or large strides. And it is not only our legs on the ground which move. We move our mouths as we talk, our hands as we speak, our backs as we shift in our chairs, our minds as we think. So the kind of movement I think the Wood sieve is likely to retain must have some quality of energy and force. If, therefore, my patient arrives quietly and moves silently this may point me elsewhere amongst the elements, or at the very least to the outer areas on the rim of the Wood circle where Wood may touch on elements around it which have a need to express themselves less energetically. Thoughts, too, may express themselves by their quickness or their slowness, decisions, a prime activity of the Wood element, be arrived at quickly or slowly, directions changed on a whim, words uttered speedily. But there will always be a feeling that the person likes getting on with things, getting a move-on generally.

These are all reactions which I experience and which are specific to me and to nobody else, but there will be some common factors which unite all the reactions to our encounter with the Wood element in others. To all these different ways of experiencing Wood's energy in another we will each bring our individual responses, which will have their balanced and their unbalanced aspects, as will what we are responding to. So how I respond, whilst being an attempt to define another person, also tells me a lot about me. The sieves are not mass-produced, with standard-sized holes, but are punched by me in the different sizes I have devised to make some sense of all the information streaming towards me from another.

What, then, have I brought here of my own which another person might not have needed to bring to the encounter? Definitely that first moment of recoil is something personal to me, that dislike of being pushed and my desire immediately to push back. Others might respond simply by engaging quite easily in the tit-for-tat I described earlier rather than feeling as though they are being pushed into doing something, as I do. Yet others, less easily, might find this push intimidating, making them draw back in fear; and there will be those, too, who may not even notice the push, their minds occupied with other things.

Since we are discussing this in the context of helping acupuncturists in their diagnosis, we have to take account of how far our own elemental make-up is here coming into play. In the examples I have given, it may be our own Wood element which enjoys the tit-for-tat exchange, our Water element that finds it threatening, our Metal element that rises so far above it as to find it too insignificant to notice, or our Fire element which smiles slightly at the encounter. But it is still the same expression in that other person to which our different elemental structures are responding; it is just that we perceive it through our own angles of vision. We must therefore take care not to interpret the expressions of the Wood element in the other person as having mainly to do with the Metal, Water or Fire elements in them, but see instead that it is we who are throwing shadows over the person in front of us coming from our own elements.

I am describing here merely one hypothetical encounter between the Wood element as it appears in another and me, and we can see from all the complex interactions which my description can only hint at how infinitely varied will be our individual responses to the unique combinations of elemental expressions with which each person approaches another. We should therefore never be surprised at how difficult it is to pinpoint the nature of the elements expressed in our patients, and give ourselves sufficient time to do this, rather than chiding ourselves for labouring so long at the task.

CHAPTER 8

FURTHER RESPONSES TO THE ELEMENTS
Earth Five Meetings

My reaction to the Wood element differs very widely from how I experience the presence of the Fire element, where my first response is far from the recoil and then the counter-movement with which I meet Wood. Here that inner smile I was describing as one of my reactions to Wood, but normally a somewhat delayed one, a kind of after-taste it leaves behind in me, shifts its position to the fore, and becomes my first reaction, for Fire is looking for just that response from me and is delighted when I respond in kind. We noted that Wood wanted to create space around it in which it could move forward. Fire always likes to have somebody occupying that space, and tries to draw those around into this space with its smile. People is what Fire is about, where we can describe Wood as about action.

I see Wood as the single bud on the bough, occupied with its own need to expand and open up; Fire, with Wood's actions to build upon, now has the leisure to look around itself and see its neighbouring buds upon that bough. Buds in nature have their own individual presence, and, if we were to draw them, we would show each with an individual, clearly-defined outline. When summer's heat unfolds them to their full extent, the borders of one bud flow into the next so that a tree in full bloom loses its individual sharp edges and fuses itself together into a greater whole. From afar, the profusion of fully-opened buds together creates a swathe of a single colour, the trees all in green, flowers and shrubs in multicoloured abundance, all appearing to lose some of their individuality as they cluster together and their outlines meld into one another. This is just an illusion, for viewed close at hand we can still see each individual leaf and flower, yet the picture as a whole helps us understand how nature, drawn outwards and upwards by the heat of the sun, stretches out in as wide an arc as it can. This image is a good illustration of Fire's need to extend beyond itself to reach out to others and meld with them. And this provides some explanation for my reactions when I am in its presence in my fellow human beings.

With Fire I have the added complication that it is my own guardian element, and therefore I have a particular resonance with its manifestations in other people. It is always difficult for us to disentangle what comes from us and what comes from others, and the differing needs we all express will act upon each other and have the potential to distort our perceptions if we are not very careful. Since each practitioner has a particular resonance with their own element, a similar process occurs for all of us in the presence of whatever element is our own, and I will use the Fire element, with my association with it, as illustration of what is a general principle. This can be stated, a bit whimsically and baldly, as 'Beware your own element, and the traps it sets for you and your patients.'

One particular trap for me is the desire to see any warmth I detect in others as a reflection of their dominant Fire element, rather than a reflection either of mine, because I will be trying so hard to draw warmth out of others, or of another's joy in basking in my warmth. Here we must remember that all the elements are within all of us, creating the whole range of physical and emotional expressions of our being, and, in the case of the Fire element, we obviously all have a heart which beats to keep us alive and is warmed emotionally by another's warmth. So the warmth within us will be stirred a little to life by that of another, but will not be sustained for as long or in the same way unless it encounters a similar expression coming from the dominant emotion in another person.

I must therefore pay particular attention to the feelings I experience within myself in the presence of Fire as another's guardian element. I have found that one way this expresses itself within me is in a warm glow continuing long after the initial contact has finished. It is as though my whole being relaxes a little, and allows itself to bask in another's warmth, as some of the endless need to warm others, which is my task, is handed over for a brief time to someone else. A fellow practitioner, observing me with patients, told me once, to my initial surprise, that I looked completely different when I was with a Fire patient. It is as though the two of us are having a kind of secret party, he said, to which he, whose guardian element was not Fire, felt rather like an uninvited guest, excluded somewhat from the general merriment. The stoking up of two fires, as it were, initially warmed him, then left him slightly shrivelled, as though they had burnt too brightly and temporarily scorched him. So where I feel a relaxing inside me, as though in a familiar presence, others may feel slightly less comfortable, more wary, as they experience the glow of Fire as too hot and immediate.

And there is another side to this. In me, too, this first feeling of welcome relaxation may be followed by a kind of inner withdrawal, for I may then start to become aware, not only of the warmth Fire brings with it, but of its needs, and these may so echo mine as to make me somewhat uneasy, as I struggle not to allow them inappropriate expression. I might be tempted to allow too close an intimacy, reflecting that party atmosphere my fellow acupuncturist noticed, where I might overstep the boundaries which enable me as practitioner to observe my patient with the necessary detachment a professional relationship demands. So a kind of tension may arise within me as I watch my reactions carefully, on the alert for any signs that I am allowing myself to respond more closely than I should to whatever echo within myself my patient evokes.

The reverse of this need for slight wariness is my familiarity with the needs my Fire patients express, and thus the possibility, if I gauge things properly, of setting up a good relationship and preparing the ground for good treatment more quickly than I may do in the presence of other elements. Fire, too, more unwilling to take than to give, will not wish to dwell long upon its miseries and will try to make light of what to other elements may be heavy burdens. If, then, I observe myself mimicking this by allowing my patient to encourage me to shrug off the seriousness of what I am being told by accepting at face value statements such as, 'Oh well, this is nothing compared with what other people have to go through', I have to stop, and take stock by reminding myself of my tendency to do the same myself, knowing, as I do, that at heart I dearly want to hear the person I am talking to say something like, 'Yes, but that does not make your own troubles any the less.'

The direction of the pull Fire exercises upon me is therefore not quite as clear as that of the Wood element. It will not wish to draw anything from me, preferring instead to offer me something, and yet I may find this offering disturbing for its very warmth or for its similarity to what I offer, and then want to withdraw a little to give myself more space. Each element in its desire to express its needs demands some reaction from us, and for each of us these demands will be at differing levels, depending upon our own overall state of balance, and particularly of the balance of our guardian element. And yet we must not attempt to brush out our personal reactions to another by denying they are there. Rather, we must learn to assess their true value as always being significant, and in so doing accept that in that assessment must be included some proper appraisal of any inevitable personal bias coming from us. Then we are able to make true use of our own interactions in helping us diagnose those of others.

I have a slightly less complicated relationship with Earth than I have with Fire, for it is not my element, but a slightly more complicated one than I have with Wood. The physical space it demands may appear not too challenging, but it is with the emotional space it asks of me that I have more trouble. I have had to do quite a lot of work on myself to gain a proper perspective on this element's presence in others, for I find it can have the capacity to irritate me in some way. And when I have tried to trace this irritation to its source, I arrive at the conclusion, painful as it originally was to me, that I am envious of Earth's ability unashamedly, in my eyes, to demand what I hesitate to demand for myself, but, I realize, would dearly like to demand. I find that somewhere inside me there is a much more needy child longing to be fed and mothered and looked after than I care ever to admit to, and when these very Earth-type needs are expressed by others I can feel exasperated, and almost affronted, by the sheer nakedness of the needs expressed, even though the expression of Wood's equally naked need, as I see it, to forge a way forward leaves me much less personally touched. I now recognize that first moment of being pulled at as though sucked slightly forwards by some centrifugal force exerted by the Earth needs of another as an expression of its need to demand nourishment of me at all levels, followed always by an inner recoil within me as I suppress my irritation at such an overt expression of a need I feel inappropriate to express myself.

But I can also sometimes experience a slight feeling of rejection in the presence of Earth, as though I am in the presence of a slightly disgruntled person who is not getting what they want and petulantly pushes me away because they feel their need is not being answered, a kind of 'see if I care' sort of a gesture. And then there is also a different kind of pressure upon me, which is as though I am being offered something I don't want, much as though an Earth person is forcing some food on me against my wishes and I try to turn away, as a child turns its head away to avoid eating food it doesn't like. And the food here might be to me an inappropriate offering of sympathy, Earth's emotion. One of my Earth patients, coming as the last person at the end of the day, commiserated with me, saying 'You poor dear, working so hard. You must be tired after such a long day, and you still have me to treat!' This initially surprised me, for I was not tired. And then I realized that what she was in effect saying behind the words was, 'Oh poor me! What if Nora hasn't got enough left to pay me the attention I need?' Here, behind the push at me, which I experienced as an imposition of inappropriate concern placed upon me, there was the hidden pull of 'I need something, too. Please give it to me, however tired you are.'

In the presence both of Fire and Earth I therefore experience a slightly stronger personal reaction than I do with the other three elements. With the next element along the cycle, Metal, I experience the least cause of all to arm myself against my own potentially unbalanced needs, and the greatest ease at recognizing within it something which adds to me rather than takes away from me. And this makes Metal the simplest element for me to work with, provided, and this is a big proviso, that I recognize its presence in good time and adapt promptly to that recognition. For, of all the elements, it will assess immediately whether or not I am responding appropriately, and, if I am, relax within a respectful space where the two of us each accept the other for what we are. The movement within me is again one of moving back, as it was with Wood, but in quite another way. It is not in the nature of a recoil to avoid what I experience as a push, but more to allow space between us in which the two of us can move without in any way impeding the other. With Earth, we are asked to be involved and thus appear very hands-on.

With Metal, on the other hand, we must be very hands-off, so far hands-off that we can be in danger of detaching ourselves completely, almost to the point of wondering why Metal patients need to come for treatment since they do so much of the work themselves and appear to demand so little of us. But, and this is the big condition, that little they demand is very specific and focused, and has to be met as perfectly as possible by our response.

For, to Metal, to appear inadequate is the thing it fears the most, and it will always at heart regard its acceptance of the need to have treatment as a kind of failure to solve its own problems by itself. The very act of turning to others for help will appear a form of admission of its own imperfection, and, since one of its needs is to attempt to achieve perfection, to get things right, this means that the act of approaching each treatment bears a strain within it alien to the other elements. If, as practitioners, we acknowledge this to be so by allowing our Metal patients to dictate the course of treatment more than we may do with the other elements, we are responding appropriately to Metal's need to forge its own path as far as possible by itself, with only the slightest nudge from us to keep it on track. And this makes for a very delicate interaction between us. I am therefore aware of the need to keep some space between me and my Metal patients, more space than with any other element. I must try to provide a kind of no-go area for myself which allows Metal to work out its own solutions without what would appear to it to be the demeaning spectacle of their practitioner observing every stage of this work.

With our final element, Water, however, things are very different, for Water, desiring to immerse itself in that greater whole, just as winter draws back into the womb of nature, draws us in with it, needing the comfort and reassurance of our presence at every stage of our interaction with them. This drawing of us towards it has something in it of the nature of

Earth's pull, but is more diffuse and less focused, revealing
a more generalized need to have all things, including me,
circling around it, rather than Earth's more specific need to
have me, in particular, drawn towards it to feed it. But we
may not feel comfortable in ourselves as we confront this
final one of the basic needs of the five elements, for, as we
know, fear lies at the heart of Water, and fear unsettles us all.
So with Water I feel jittery in myself without quite knowing
why, for the fears and anxieties it feels emanate from it in
often hidden ways, since to show them, and thus to make
itself more vulnerable, is what it strives hardest to avoid. I
am aware of some inner jerkiness in myself, an unsettled
feeling of pressure upon me coming from I know not where.
This is far from the precise, focused pressure I experience
with Wood which confronts me head-on. It is much more
difficult to pinpoint the direction of Water's pressure, almost
as though I am immersed (such a Water-like word!) in a field
of subtle anxieties and buffeted by waves on all sides. I am
always aware of the force Water exerts upon me as it seeks
to move wherever it wants, without regard for anything else,
much as though a torrent or an avalanche may be lurking to
be unleashed against all it encounters at any moment.

I will observe in myself two kinds of reaction. I will observe
that I am attempting to calm something that is disturbed; my
hands seem to want to stretch themselves out in front of me,
palms down, as though I am pressing them down to still some
agitation. This is the gesture we all make if we attempt to
defuse a difficult situation, a 'come on now, let's all take things
easily, there's no need for all this trouble' kind of gesture. It
is a kind of pacifying, calming movement, as though I am
trying, again using appropriate Water terminology, to pour
oil on troubled waters. The other reaction I have observed
in myself is that I find myself murmuring along with my
patient, as if we are singing a kind of gentle duet together,
which is unlike the to-and-fro of everyday conversation where

one person waits for the other to finish before replying. I appear to be responding to the fear in my patient's voice which lies behind the words spoken rather than to what is actually being said. I am thus providing a kind of calming accompaniment, almost subliminally accepted by both as being necessary, so that the fact that we are in a way talking over each other is secondary to the comfort the reassuring murmur I am offering gives my patient. Here the content of what is said becomes secondary to the underlying message the patient is conveying to me, which is of a deep-lying fear, and to the underlying message I am responding with, which is a reassurance that all will be well.

A further indication of interest in assessing which element we are dealing with is the amount of physical or emotional space we are asked to leave between us and our patient. With Wood, I feel I am being pushed aside, as Wood tries to forge ahead and past me. With Fire, the space between us is more fluid. It does not want me to come too close to it before it has decided how it wants to approach me, but will approach me warmly of its own volition when it feels safe to do so. I must not, however, try to keep it close to me longer than it wants, for, though enjoying the warmth of all encounters, it will also find their closeness an area of potential conflict peculiar to itself and to no other element, since the field of relationships is where it may have to do battle, and all relationships harbour within them the potential to hurt the heart deep within the Fire element. So the space between my Fire patients and me needs a more delicate form of adjustment than that between Wood and me, for Wood is not as concerned as Fire is with its personal interactions or with the intricacies of working out exactly what emotional space it is comfortable with. With Earth I enter a much more comfortable physical space into which I am as though pulled, though this, too, as we have seen, brings its own complications with it. With Metal I must make sure that I do not intrude into its precious space with inappropriately quick or disturbing interventions. Finally, Water will demand that I move closer to it, as I find myself trying to calm and pacify it, as though through my own stillness I will still turbid waters.

In all these examples of the emotional and physical spaces within which I act out my encounters with others, I have drawn upon the many, many interactions over the years which have gradually enabled me to fill out my own personal template of the pull or push each of the elements exerts upon me. As I have said, others will experience the elements differently, because each of us has developed our own individual responses. What is important in all this is to see how necessary for making accurate diagnoses it is to be very self-aware, for it is on the accuracy of this self-awareness that much of the accuracy of our diagnoses rests. There is no truer use of the dictum 'know thyself', and such knowledge comes free! But it is often derided because, in the final analysis, it cannot be found in books, not even in this one, for all book learning must refer at the deepest level back to what is in ourselves and what we already at heart know, but often choose to ignore.

CHAPTER 9

Conversations with the Elements
Exchange Pledges

From where, within each one of us, do these expressions of the elements arise which culminate in the step forward or the step back I take, mentally or physically, in the presence of the energies of another person? Something is pouring out from this person (and pouring out is not too strong a description), which impacts so strongly upon me that I am compelled into movement, sometimes against my will. The placatory gestures Water may summon from me, the space I move back into to allow Metal its own, the comforting embrace Earth calls me to give it, are all stimulated from within these other people out there, demanding some response from me which without these demands I would not feel drawn to give. It is not enough in this context simply to say that this is how these people are expressing their needs. From an acupuncture perspective we need to know what is actually happening to the energies within that one or other person which is expressing itself as a particular need, for, if that expression is unbalanced, we have to pinpoint the origin of that imbalance, and its degree, in order to work out what treatment is required to redress it.

It is not too fanciful to think of the different kinds of pressures exerted by the elements upon me as different types of a kind of conversation I have with the organs deep inside my patients, to be interpreted in just as specific terms as if they had addressed me in words. To use another analogy, we also enter into a kind of dance with each person we meet, as we adjust, sometimes subtly, sometimes more roughly, what we want of them to what they want of us. In acupuncture terms, the adjustment must be much more on my part than on my patient's, for my aim is to see them as they are, not for them to feel the need to change to fit in with my needs (although, sadly, it may well happen that we do not achieve this high aim every time, in our clumsiness forcing our patients sometimes to do the adjusting). But it is nonetheless a dance, a kind of a two-step, in which I at times try to follow my patient's lead and at others, where I feel my patient needs guidance and direction, take the lead.

As the elements in my patients move towards ever greater balance as treatment progresses, the pressures they place on my interaction with them alters, and I have to be sensitive and flexible enough to adapt to these changes in our relationship. And since it is how we together manoeuvre the intricacies of the relationship between us which dictates the course, and ultimately the success, of treatment, it should not be surprising that I devote so much of this discussion to the tricky questions these relationships give rise to. This is where too little work is often done by us, but so much needs to be done. For the selection of a specific treatment is the end-point of a process which starts within the patient at each day of treatment, and spreads out from the patient to me as the elements within him/her send out their messages of today towards me. It then continues within me as I attempt to decipher these messages with the help of my own elements, aided by whatever skills in interpretation I have accumulated over the years, before finally passing back from me to my patient through the words I speak and through the treatment I decide upon.

The needle laid upon the skin at a specific point or points is the culmination of the process. And then we sit back, as it were, the patient and I, to await the outcome, which then feeds itself back to me at the start of the next encounter, creating a kind of spiral which draws within it any changes brought about by life or by the treatment, modifying itself to them and incorporating them into the next spin of the spiral.

The signals the elements send out change as evidence of imbalance, and change again in response to treatment, this time as evidence, we hope, of greater balance. Each treatment summons a response, not only from the element which I have selected to treat, but from all the elements, since 'one for all and all for one' is how they work, and this response may be as negative as a stony silence where nothing moves, which I interpret as a direction to turn elsewhere. Then there will be clearer responses in terms of some changes in sensory information coming from the patient, a slightly different colour, a slightly brighter eye, a hint of a smile, for example. What is happening here is that the needle has stimulated an acupuncture point, or a number of points, along a specific meridian, sending a signal along the meridian increasing its flow of energy. The stimulation will certainly run the length of the whole meridian, increasing energy within the whole area over which it passes, and it will also, more significantly because at a greater depth, thrust this increase of healthy energy inwards deep inside along the pathways which connect the exterior with the interior, until it reaches the organ itself connected to the meridian whose point we have stimulated on the surface.

The transfer of energy from the surface, as the needle touches the point, to the deep, where the organ responds, is immediate, as the whole of our organism responds as one to the change in energy the needle is effecting. I have observed this happening by feeling a patient's pulses as another practitioner needles, and feeling the pulses change as the needle connects with the point. In my own treatments I can feel my mouth curve into an involuntary smile as soon as points are needled which stimulate my Fire energy and thus convey the joy it craves, as healthy energy passing from my

Heart and Small Intestine meridians on the surface warms the heart itself deep within. I do not feel this if points on other meridians are stimulated or if somebody tries to give me a placebo treatment on a non-acupuncture point in an attempt to see whether points do what we say they do. And they do! It always feels so reassuring to me to know from my own experiences in this way that what I have learnt in theory is in practice true. I feel that I am thereby given my own personal proof that all things are indeed one, that the Dao, the All, which enfolds everything, enfolds me, too, in its grasp, and thus that every time I apply my understanding of my practice to the treatments I offer, I am re-establishing or strengthening further the knots which tie us all into what is.

We are fortunate in that nature is kind to us, and does not appear to want to punish us, except with a silence, if we are not addressing the elements where their need shows. It is very rare, indeed I think it is almost impossible, for treatment to make a condition worse, or make a patient feel worse, except perhaps temporarily, as a warning sign that our attempt to change the quality of the flow of energy in some way is not directed in the right quarter. There may be a brief feeling of discomfort, of something not being quite right after such treatments, but this appears soon to be balanced out by the patient's own attempts to keep their energies flowing correctly. It seems that we have some kind of self-regulating mechanism within us which prevents the acupuncturist from going too far astray, and which encourages the patient's energies to protect themselves. It is as though they do not allow us to interfere too much against what they feel is their proper flow, and only permit the longer-term interference from our needles if that interference is in line with what they feel is a balanced need.

In fact, I suspect that it takes quite a lot of pressure in the first place to turn what is balanced within us into what is unbalanced, and this works in our favour if the treatment we have selected is not contributing to the balance we hoped it would, but instead is further pushing awry something already slightly or strongly out of kilter. There have been numerous occasions on which my treatment has initially not been directed where it should because my senses have not been honed sufficiently to give me accurate feedback, and thus my assessment of what the patient's elements need is somewhat faulty, but there have certainly not been anywhere near as many occasions when my patients appear to have been affected in any detrimental way by such treatment or have complained about it. Far from it. Often it is I who have been dissatisfied with what treatment is achieving, not my patient, who may be less impatient than I am, for they certainly do not know, as I do, how startling can eventually be the changes towards greater health once I have directed treatment where it needs to go.

The danger here is that treatment may instead circle round on itself, if it changes nothing, a form of 'vicious circle', but without the viciousness implied in the term. Perhaps a form of ultimately sterile circling would be a better expression, for if treatment turns round and round, as though moving along the same circular tramlines, it can only reinforce rather than redress an imbalance. The aim must be to move the patient forward out of the kind of ruts imbalances can create, and the jolt the needle gives to the energy, stimulating it to change, is then like the jolt we give somebody or something to free it from what can feel like helpless entrapment within an unchanging situation. And change, sometimes, we feel, any change, is better than being stuck, like a poor mouse on its wheel, treading the same rungs round and round and going precisely nowhere.

But in what direction does the patient need to go? It is not really a question of any change being better than none, though initially this may be true. Once jolted out of an imbalance, a patient has to move in a different direction, and who is to decide exactly what this is? And here we return to the elements, and to the patient's guardian element, for as it gains greater balance it glimpses a path ahead which is already laid down for it, but which in its imbalance it has lost sight of. Once this element achieves greater balance, each treatment is then like an axe cutting away tangled growth and revealing the way forward, pointing the patient towards the development of the full potential of their guardian element. It is then that patients start telling me, often in strikingly similar words, things like, 'Now I know who I am', or 'Now I know where I am going', or, 'Now I feel more myself than I have ever done.' This shows that, deep inside each of us, there is a voice telling us that we do indeed know who we are and where we should be going, if we can only hear it above the strident noises going on around us which often seem to be trying to shout us down and push us in directions we don't want to go.

To me this is the most comforting and at the same time awe-inspiring aspect of my work – that revealed to me through it is evidence that there is a potential within each of us, which, if realized, leads directly deep inside to a unique core within us, which is the 'I' that has been decreed for us since our conception, or, who knows, even before that. It always feels to me to be such a privilege to be allowed to work at this level with my patients, and to be paid for it! Sometimes I feel it should be I who pay my patients for being granted permission to enter such sacred ground with them.

What is always heartening is to appreciate the extent to which we are given at any moment the opportunity to change if we wish to do so throughout our life. The only thing that remains constant appears to be that solid, unique inner core which determines who we are, but how this inner core expresses itself is as subject to the endless processes of change as our outer, physical structure housing this core is subject to. Just as we slough off our body's tissues cell by cell in a process of constant renewal, as one dying cell is replaced by another living cell in the intricate manoeuvres which move each tiniest part of us forward on its way from the start of its life to the last stages of the ageing process, so we slough off that deepest part of us, our inner being, layer by layer, in a process of endless transformation.

At any stage in this journey of life, some mischance may occur which impedes one or other part of us from unfolding and replicating itself in this balanced process of renewal, causing a hitch in what, in balance, should be the smooth, uninterrupted and thus imperceptible, processes of change. If we liken this to the development of the rings of growth on a tree trunk, then it is as though some slight obstacle has inserted itself within one of these circling rings, causing it to deviate slightly from its harmonious, spiralling ascent. And such a deviation will appear on the outside of the trunk initially as a slight bump, and then, if serious enough, as a malformation which pulls the straight trunk out of alignment. It is a similar such process which occurs in the spiralling, circling movement of the elements around our central core.

CHAPTER 10

The Elements under Stress
Not at Ease

I am writing this at the height of the credit crunch in 2009, when much that once appeared safe has almost overnight become unstable, as though the very ground under our feet has shifted in some cataclysmic earthquake. We can no longer be sure that many of the things we took so long for granted can still be relied upon, something I am aware of each time I walk past the closed shutters of our local Woolworths, and experience a tiny jolt of fear at the disappearance of this pillar of the high street. Insecurity rules, bringing with it an all-pervasive undertow of fear, a feeling that events are no longer under human control. This has made me think again about how individual elements react to stresses such as these, for they place a great burden upon them, and the elements' need to work together becomes increasingly important.

How such stresses affect each of us will vary markedly depending upon our view of life, our innate sense of optimism or pessimism, our love of adventure or of stability, our fear of the uncertain or our flexibility to change, and ultimately on the kind of balance our elements, and in particular our guardian element, provide us with. Whenever we are under stress of any kind the elements start to reveal themselves in their true colours, because pressure upon them brings their individual characteristics into starker relief than does a more even-tempered flow of life. The greater the stress, then, the more visible become the characteristic signatures a particular element stamps upon us. It is therefore useful to look at how each element reacts to stress, as another way of deepening our perceptions of the different characteristics of the elements. This in turn will help us in our diagnoses.

So let us first look at the Wood element. We know that one of Wood's characteristics is to demand order, to ask that things take their proper place in the scheme of things in an ordered universe. When that order is threatened, as it is now, this is likely to increase Wood's need to feel it has to be in control of things, or at the very least to know that others are taking steps to bring them under control. Wood's emotion, a forcefulness which we call anger, can then become exaggerated, as the greater sense of chaos in the world around it puts additional pressure upon its need to feel that order is maintained. Where there is insufficient balance in a person's Wood element, then, it will try to overcompensate by showing an increased need for greater control of all aspects of its life, even the most trivial, and, of course, in heightened expressions of anger.

This might take the form of an increasingly authoritarian approach to life, with the laying down of rigid rules which it will try to impose not only on itself but more often on others. It may therefore become more inflexible in its thinking and in its actions, the emotional equivalent of a tightening of our physical tendons and ligaments, the parts of the body over which it has control. It believes that this increased rigidity is a way of forcing order upon what it regards as the chaotic unravelling of life.

Fire will have quite different reactions. It is a more flexible element, in some respects the most flexible of all in certain conditions. Its playful, taking-life-as-it-comes, side can come to the fore here, as can its enjoyment of the sheer excitement which can be created at times of stress, as its natural yang exuberance is stimulated by the heightened tension in the air. It will also always try to find reasons for humour, as a way of warming its own and others' hearts, and excels in the kind of macabre glee dire events can evoke. On the other hand, of course, any stress may accentuate its imbalances, and then it will lose some of its ability to try to look on the sunny side of life, as it starts to feel it is under threat. It will try to shrug off its insecurities as long as it can, succumbing only when it starts to lose its ability to remain positive.

Fire's daughter element, Earth, will not so much look for action as for support in times of crisis, seeking comfort in the presence of others. One of its greatest needs is to reassure itself that its responsibilities are shared and thus some of its burdens lifted by others. In the current stressful times, it will take comfort from feeling that decisive action has been taken by others. Any imbalance will reveal itself in a more determined effort to hunker down and tuck itself in, to ensure it is surrounded by others. It will feel it can cope if it doesn't feel alone, needing the company of others, of anybody, no matter who, provided that these others do not demand too much of it and therefore threaten to take rather than to give. It has a surprising ability to shut its eyes to what it does not want to see, in an effort to convince itself that what is disturbing out there need not affect it. Perhaps of all the elements it is the one that needs most to protect itself from any level of disturbance which might upset its need for the warm comforts of a safe home in which to shelter, avoiding as long as possible having to admit the existence of anything that shakes these foundations.

Metal, on the other hand, seeks not the shelter and comfort Earth craves, but the space in which to contemplate what is happening and to assess what its reactions to this should be. Its detachment can give it a strength the other elements can lack, for it can to some extent maintain, sometimes against all the odds, that the events around it need not affect it, as though it builds a gap between these and itself. Its ability to find perspective helps it put the most tragic and far-reaching events into a wider context than may other, more immediately engaged, elements.

Its imbalances, as with those of all the other elements, will of course weaken this ability, and reduce the distance it tries to maintain between itself and what is going on around it. And then it can no longer draw so successfully on its ability to observe events with the detachment other elements admire. It is likely that its own perception of this failure will increase its already dominant yin qualities, so that it may become increasingly passive and introspective. Depression, so appropriate a term for the feeling we all experience at events pressing down too hard upon us, is a particularly apt description of Metal's unbalanced response here, as it sinks lower under the weight of its inability to stand to one side as it would like to.

Finally we come to Water, of all elements the most likely to respond initially with panic, because of its dominant emotion, fear, and then, when it is sufficiently balanced, to find within itself the strength not only to float along with events and not be overwhelmed by them, but to swim against their tide and survive come what may. Its first reaction will always be that of a startled rabbit caught in the headlights of a fast approaching car, and this fear brings with it the rush of adrenalin described in Western medical terms as our fight or flight reflex. It will try first to flee, and when this proves no longer possible it will turn to fight, and fight to the death if necessary. There is no more vicious a fighter than a cornered Water person. If anybody is to escape the chaos of destructive events it will be Water, for it knows how to be ruthless at the expense of others, a ruthlessness often necessarily disguised so that its opponents have no time to work out ways of countering it. But the possibility of panic is always there close to the surface, threatening to overwhelm it and undermine its ability to work out ways of surviving, and then in its imbalance it can indeed come close to drowning.

The qualities I describe here are, of course, necessarily more stereotyped than they will appear in any individual person, and since we are formed of all the elements in some unique combination, no one person of any particular element will show the characteristics of this element under stress exactly as I have described them in such stark outline. They will always be shaded by the individual idiosyncracies which shape us. It is nonetheless always useful to try to lay down a general elemental framework within which to attempt to fit people.

One of the most useful tools to help us trace the elements is to look for places and times when people are particularly likely to show themselves under stress, and these are likely to be when they gather together and we can watch them interact with one another. This will be particularly so in inherently stressful situations, such as a city rush-hour or a long queue at the supermarket checkout. I have also found watching television to be one of the best ways of seeing the elements in all their nakedness, with radio a close second, or a definite first if we are trying to define a person's tone of voice. People reveal their true natures in situations such as the news which by its very nature forces them to show themselves as themselves, since being in the limelight places everybody under stress. Here we are likely to see the grieving father, the frightened asylum seeker or the angry neighbour in stark colours, since interviews are necessarily kept short to retain an audience's limited attention span, and will have been chosen precisely with the object of showing the most telling and revealing aspects of a situation. This is when we are most likely to see the elements in sharp relief, the grieving, the frightened and the angry person showing more heightened expressions of their grief, fear and anger than normal.

And then, of course, there is the inherently stressful situation which is that of the practice room itself. We often choose to overlook this, believing as we do that we should be providing a loving, caring environment for our patients where stress is avoided as much as possible. Loving and caring it may and should be, but this does not mean that it is not also stressful in its own way, for it is in this room that the patient is put under the kind of pressure from close and acute questioning which will help to accentuate the characteristics of their individual elements in a way which should help, not hinder, treatment.

Having decided that help is needed, and that we, as practitioners, are the ones they are entrusting with the responsibility of helping them, patients have to confront the fears which any self-exposure is likely to arouse in even the bravest of us. And some form of self-exposure, some opening up of doors to our inner self which we might prefer to remain closed, forms part of any therapeutic work, and is implicit in the kind of questioning which will lead to our diagnosis. To reveal intimate thoughts and hopes in itself places a stress all its own upon the elements, and as acupuncturists we frequently see our patients made uncomfortable by probing questioning. Here the elements can start to reveal themselves in all their nakedness, throwing up clear diagnostic signals indicating their presence. With increasing experience we can learn ways of drawing the elements out into the open in this way, but not in such a way as to alarm the patient. A delicate balance has to be drawn between acceptable probing and offensive intrusion.

For the practitioner, too, the practice room will provide its own stresses, and all of us should be aware of how our own guardian element is likely to affect or even interfere with treatment. I have already discussed the particular pressures the patient/practitioner encounter will bring with it, and practitioners, like patients, may feel vulnerable and defensive, and, if not acknowledging this to themselves, allow the elements within them also to cast their own distorting shadows over the patient.

Obviously there are many other ways in which we can watch the elements at work, and we have to find those which we feel offer us the deepest insights into the different characteristics of the elements. We must always, however, remember that continued hard work is required of us to keep the elements before us, and not to grow lazy and think we now know enough. So complex are the skills needed to unravel the tangled, interlocking skeins of the elements that we can never be complacent. These are skills we need to hone every day, much as a tennis player or a marathon runner has to train daily to remain in good condition. It is all too easy to become lazy, and just regard our practice room as the only place where we need to practise.

CHAPTER 11

THE LINE BETWEEN BALANCE AND IMBALANCE

Heavenly Pivot

It is comparatively simple to write in very general terms about the marks the individual elements imprint upon us. We can say the sound of a Fire voice is laughing, or the colour of Earth is yellow, and this is accurate as far as it goes. Unfortunately, it doesn't go very far, since we are not composed of just one element, but of all of them in differing combinations, each element colouring the next within us to create a unique blend which represents me rather than you, and distinguishes the person on my right from the person on my left. We can therefore never actually see the elements in their individual glory, but always tinged with shades of the other elements, making recognition of what is the dominant shading in any of the sensory marks upon us no easy task. We need all the help that we can get in this, and it is always a slow, laborious business, which never comes to an end, because just as we think we have mastered one of these aspects, perhaps thinking that we can now distinguish the laughing from the singing voice, a person comes along who puts our new-found skill to the test by apparently being of the Fire element and yet not having the kind of laughing voice we thought he should have. And then we are forced to acknowledge that our understanding of the different shadings has to go a little deeper still, for each person weaves a dense pattern of sensory information as our elements together engage within us in their unique dance of creation.

It is always good to refer back to nature to help underpin our understanding, because nature reflects the work of the elements in their cosmic simplicity much more purely and directly, and in the least complicated way. I imagine that when I say the words spring or autumn, they evoke in all of us clear-cut images of buds on trees or the splendour of burnished leaves. There is, of course, a strong echo of these simple pictures when we think of their equivalents in us, but unfortunately here the image is overlaid with more confusing layers, for the buds in a Wood person do not exist on their own. In spring, buds can be said to be visible expressions of the energies which the Wood element breathes into the trees. The seeds from which they came, the blossom into which they will grow, the fruit which they will produce and the dryness of the dying leaves have no place here until they come into season and their time is right. In the human being, on the other hand, within the buds of Wood are present always the seed, the blossom, the fruit and the decaying leaves, which the other elements are there to work on, for within us are all the organs as their expressions. Our Water, Fire, Earth and Metal elements may not dominate in spring, but they do not abdicate their responsibility or fade into nothing as their equivalents in nature do. Since they still have an essential part to play in the energetic system which creates a Wood person, their signatures remain strong, and can often confuse us into thinking one or other is dominant, and the colourings they give to the Wood element modify and often obscure the buds lying deep within. This is as though the branch bears not only buds but leaves in full bloom, fruit hanging from it and the dying splendour of leaves in autumn, all mixed together.

To ask nature to help us detect the presence of Wood as the dominant element in a person, though in itself an essential and helpful part of our diagnosis, is therefore unfortunately not helpful enough. Human beings are much more complex than any tree. Dissect a tree, and we find simplicity itself.

Dissect a human being, and we find instead layer upon layer of intricate, deeply varied structures, and each of these, as they develop functions of their own, modify this structure, and, in element terms, add their own patina to the overall colouring. Their very differences have the potential to draw our eyes away from the whole to its parts, as they can do if we are not careful.

At the heart of this whole, this five-fold cluster of elements, each creating and shaping the physical organs within us, lies the core of each person's individuality, their guardian element. In trying to disentangle from this skein of interlocking energies the one which gives the complex pattern its unique imprint, we have to learn to grade the elements in terms of their importance, and this is where the difficulty lies. How often, for example, have we taken the laugh covering up the fear as evidence of Fire rather than Water as the dominant element, or the yellow covering up the white as evidence of the Earth rather than the Metal element? We have to assess each of the sensory signals in turn, and having attempted to grade them, we then have to compare them, for they must together finally point to one element, however much the others, too, are involved.

We have, too, to assess which of the five elements are showing themselves as being in balance and which are not. And here we come to the tricky question as to what exactly, in terms of health of body and soul, we can call balance and what imbalance. It may well be, to confuse matters further, that just as the saying goes, 'One man's meat may be another man's poison', so may one man's (or woman's) balance be another's imbalance. For all is, and must remain, relative, relative to that person at that stage in their life and with those stresses to deal with and those challenges to confront. I have argued elsewhere (*Keepers of the Soul*) that we are, as I put it, necessarily incomplete, that our element's challenges need not, indeed should not, be regarded as something prejudicial to us, to be overcome and set aside as soon as we can, but instead as forming a necessary part of the spiral of human development, creating a constantly evolving potential if we choose to view it in these terms, or, if we do not, as a constant irritation, a burden we view as irksome. I will continue to argue this as long as I have breath to do so, and pen to write, for I can see no other reason for the continuing evolution of the human being towards ever more complex forms. Here I think of a six-year-old's ability to grasp the details of a computer or a mobile phone in a few minutes which I, at 70, struggle helplessly with. And because the brain continues to evolve in this way, it will soon have devised robots to do so much of our work that we will have time to be ever more creative.

If a state of balance is neither possible, nor, in human terms, even ultimately desirable, our assessment of how far any particular element needs support from our treatment will always be a very subjective one. This assessment must take account of our understanding that all beings and all things are constantly in process of development, or, as I put it, pass through different stages of becoming. Our physical body provides such a clear example of this that it is odd that we ever query this fact, as by implication we often do in Western medical terms, when we believe that a blood sample or tissue biopsy or a BP reading, taken at any one point will remain the same a few minutes later, let alone a few weeks later. The line between balance and imbalance is therefore always a fluid one, and can never be definitively drawn, and many factors have to be taken into account before we judge that signals from the elements are balanced or not. Thus for one person a high red colour may not indicate the imbalance in Fire we think it is, but instead show that the person is happy!

In acupuncture, the concept of energy ever on the move is so fundamental a part of all we do that we assume that each treatment we offer must alter something and continue to do so, rather than, as in the West, being regarded as something having a fixed, finite aim, the lowering of blood pressure or the elimination of migraine, for example. From our perspective, this is too static an approach, for it takes no account of the constant layers of change time places upon us, making a treatment appropriate for today totally inappropriate or ineffective for tomorrow. Thus to find ourselves endlessly repeating treatments of the same drug or the same groupings of acupuncture points goes against all that we understand to be the fluctuating, shimmering tissue of energies jostling within us and ever responding to the pressures of life within and without.

The concept of balance for any one person, too, will therefore constantly change and evolve. A patient will respond uniquely to treatment, and their responses will demand changes in the treatment schedule at each visit. This lays quite a heavy burden on all five element practitioners, and one it is often difficult to come to terms with. Even now, this need for endless flexibility, and lack of any fixed parameters within which to work and from which to take comfort, is a constant challenge to me. It would be nice, I sometimes think, if I could just 'know' before I see a patient what treatment I will give him/her that day, rather than having to wait in a kind of suspense of uncertainty for that patient to tell me, through my senses or his/her words, how I can best help and thus what today's treatment should be. It could be said that this is not a calling for the faint-hearted!

CHAPTER 12

The Tide of Fate
Dark Gate

Can I indeed always help? A question that always arises for me is the extent to which acupuncture can help stem the tide of illness and death, and therefore what I regard as the limits of what my needles can do. In theory, at least, I see no limits, although practice tells a different story, and my deep-seated belief in the power of acupuncture will be challenged from many sides, not least by my own skills. If we accept a picture of human health as being the product of a constantly self-balancing system of energetic impulses, and ill-health as the result of some malfunctioning in this system, the passage back from ill-health to health, if it is not achieved by itself, as happens when we recover spontaneously, requires the kind of intervention we have described in the previous chapters, and can obviously be achieved in many ways, and not solely by acupuncture means. There is much that can impede the restoration of health, not the least of which being what we can regard as the allotted span of an individual life, and, more mysteriously and ultimately unknowably, we can never know why this span differs so markedly from one person to the next. For instance, as I witnessed last week, we can be driving peacefully along a country road, and a tree, whipped by a storm, can uproot itself at the very moment of our passing, flinging itself down upon us and crushing the breath from us, dealing death with one apparently random throw of the dice. Or we can defy all the odds of survival in harsh conditions and yet live to be a hundred.

It may appear as though it is merely a matter of bad fortune that somebody dies at 20 whilst another reaches 80, for this implies that we lead random lives, but somewhere I like to feel, although admittedly on no evidence but my own conviction of patterns driving the universe, that there, too, chance plays little part, and all these differing spans of life have some meaning behind them. This belief of mine is often strengthened by observing how often those subjected to what could, to others, appear to be the most appalling fate, a life bound to a wheelchair, or foreshortened by illness or afflicted by tragedy, often have about them some aura, and this is not too heavy a word for it, of something deeper, indeed almost ethereal about them, as though they are touched by a kinder hand and experience deeper connections to the great beyond than those with apparently less challenged lives.

Of course, there are those whom an apparently harsh fate turns instead towards bitterness, but here again we confront the human paradox that all things that confront us in life can be viewed potentially as blessings or curses, depending on the slant of our viewpoint. I regard those prepared to accept what fate hands them, however harsh this may be, as being there in some way to teach us something. This teaching may be as simple as the ability to accept an apparently cruel fate, or as complex as placing all things in a wider context.

Looked at in this way, we have to ask whether we can indeed stem the tide of fate. If we have a certain time to live and certain burdens to bear, who am I then as acupuncturist to try and defy these odds, and how far, indeed, can I do so? Having struggled with just such conundrums since I first lifted a needle, I cannot say that I am any further along the path of finding an answer except for the simple one that I am here to do my best to help restore and maintain health and balance, as far as this is possible, and thus, in some, but not all, cases, to prolong life, again where this is possible; but that if I am presented with proof that the treatments I give are not effective in doing so, I have learnt to accept, more readily than I initially did, and now not necessarily sadly, that I am dealing here with forces greater than my own resources to counter. I say that I am not necessarily saddened by this because, as each of us has to, I have worked out my own view on this over the years, and more so as I grow older, a view of life in which death occupies an increasingly less fearful place.

I have therefore to a large extent lost my fear of a patient's dying. This was indeed a great fear initially, for it seemed to represent an absolute failure of my skills, a sign that what I regarded as life-reinforcing had encountered a hurdle it could not surmount. And in those early days, it shook my conviction that I knew what I was doing, leading to periods of great self-doubt and uncertainty. Now, viewed from a much more rounded perspective, achieved with much wrestlings of the soul, I see things differently. I do not regard my work as being a battle in which I pit my wits against the forces of ill-health harming my patients, but as something much less violent, gentler, a kind of encouragement for what is out of balance to help it return to balance, if it is in its power so to do, and, if not, a kind of gentle accompaniment along a path which may ultimately lead to death. We cannot wrench a life from the grip of death if that is what is in store for it. Where the doors of death are wide open, we can accompany a patient through them and ease their passage. However much we seek to do so, we cannot turn them aside from what lies directly ahead, though we may help a patient dally a little on the way, pick a few flowers, repair a relationship and enjoy something new and exciting. All these things we can do as we help a patient move forwards, if that is what they wish, and if our skills and understanding match sensitively our patient's needs.

And they will match them more if we accept that the struggle to maintain life has its limits, which differ for each person, and that it is not our task to define those limits, but instead to seek to recognize them for what they are. Above all, we must not be frightened to accompany our patients on this often dark and troubling path towards their death. So doing has helped me quite markedly change my own approach to these profound mysteries of life, and helped, too, my work with those less mortally sick, for it has taught me to place their disturbances and fears within a wider context, and one which helps to make more relative that which can often threaten to overbalance into some extreme. Faced with the mysteries of life's ending and the struggles it forces us often to engage in, the lesser ills take on quite a different colouring, and become gentler in tone. And this, we hope, will help us help both ourselves and our patients grade their distresses more appropriately by placing them in this wider context.

There comes a time in every life when some painful event or another forces us to try to make some sense of what has occurred, and when we try to assess the value of a life, its particular pluses or minuses. Here such phrases as, 'What has my life been about?', or 'What did I do to deserve this?', or 'Why has this happened to me?', hammer away, like some painful leitmotiv, demanding resolution. My work has forced me to look for answers to such questions since my patients have often brought with them into the practice room many stories of distress and unhappiness for which I have had to try to find a context.

Many years ago I read, to my great surprise, that the then Astronomer Royal considered that modern advances in physics had made it possible to believe that the universe might have been created specifically to pave the way for human existence. Far from our being insignificant specks in the vast and indifferent landscape of the cosmos, this places us instead at its very heart, making us significant in a way we might not have imagined. The chance of human life evolving to its current level of complexity then becomes not a thing of chance after all, but of the unimaginably intricate interweaving of many tiny occurrences all taking place simultaneously at one point in the vastness of time and one point in the vastness of space, with only one object, the creation of conditions ultimately suitable for the appearance of life. To even the most hardened of scientists not given to flights of fancy this cannot then merely be attributed to the vagaries of serendipity, but must be the result of a structured plan leading us out from the primaeval slime towards the advanced forms of human life.

These are awesome thoughts, and thoughts not for the timid, for in placing us so firmly at the centre of all things they also place a heavy responsibility upon us to act in a way which is commensurate with such a deep and challenging destiny. For all I know all this may be absurd. We may indeed only have evolved by pure chance to the level we are at now, and thus live at the whim of haphazard forces which may, at any time, snuff us out, like tiny insects squashed indifferently underfoot. On the other hand, I find it deeply satisfying to visualize my life in terms which assume a kind of human destiny far beyond that of a chance existence. I will never know, of course, whether there is a deep level of wishful thinking in this for me, for it is undoubtedly more comforting to think that life has a purpose rather than consigning it to the role of the meaningless. So what I write here is based on this perhaps improbable fact (or is it a hope?) that the universe with its precious human cargo has a direction to it, that there is an arrow moving through each individual life which points it forward to somewhere, and that somehow it is the task of this life not only to try and unravel its direction but to give to it meaning.

And this is how I try to approach the great mystery of human suffering. There is no doubt that of all living creatures we appear to be the only ones capable of suffering not merely physical pain but what I call existential pain. We have access to an inner life, the life of our soul, which, to human eyes at least, is denied most other species, except, to a limited extent, the most evolved amongst them. And whatever the view we take of human destiny, whether we think that there is such a thing as a unique human destiny, or merely a more complex destiny than those of lesser evolved animals, we cannot deny the existence of this extra dimension to human life which makes possible the development of abstract thought and the expression of emotional depth. And with such depth comes the possibility of pain, distress and dissatisfaction. In our attitude to this, and our attempt to understand why this should be so, lies the secret of what human life is all about, and with it the possibility of learning to come to terms with the tragedies as well as the joys which it hands to us.

Viewed in this way, it can seem as though some unseen force has shuffled a pack of cards and dealt us a hand not of our choosing and often not of our understanding, so confusing can the cards we are dealt seem to us. Why, for example, should one person have what appears to be a smooth life, with much happiness and no great tragedies to interrupt it, whilst another is given obstacle after obstacle to confront? Is there any sense to this? If not, how do we deal with such vagaries of fate? If there is some sense, then what meaning can or must we draw from these things to help us continue to live a productive, rather than a bitter, life?

Perhaps one way of looking at things is to think that it is the very apparent arbitrariness of the workings of our fate which lies at the heart of what our life's task is. Perhaps the attempt to make sense out of what can appear senseless has an aim all its own, making the apparently meaningless take on a meaning it is up to us to discover. Some will say that we may be inventing such a meaning, making it a figment of our imagination, to help satisfy our deep need to understand why the different steps of our individual fate have occurred when they did and in the form that they did. And who knows if they are right? For myself, it is too hard a task to attribute all to the haphazard, for I would thereby feel that I was consigning to the waste basket much of the transformative work of my life which I have felt compelled to engage in, having always a deep need to make sense out of all I experience, to transform what happens to me and around me into some pattern which adds a deeper layer to my understanding of these happenings.

Those believing in the presence of a higher being under whose control we all live may possibly be unable to understand such thoughts, for their beliefs may enable them to hand over to this higher power the burden of making sense of the inequalities of individual fate. But I cannot believe in such a solution to life's enigmas, and have had to attempt to work out my own answers in my own way.

What has brought this to the forefront of my mind has been a sequence of recent events which, taken together, have compelled me once more to confront my understanding of the part played by tragic events in the unfolding of human destiny. Three different people of my acquaintance have suffered what can only be considered the heavy blows of some uncaring fate: one the discovery of terminal cancer in a young friend of his, another a tragic compounding of already existing family woes by the sudden death of a member of the family, and the third by the equally sudden discovery of deep unhappiness in the marriage of one of her children. I had to bear witness to all these very different events, and work out my own very different reactions to each of them to enable me to offer what help and understanding I could. What I found the most difficult thing of all was how to gauge what was an appropriate response in each case and one that would not further burden those already overcome with their own sorrows. We none of us can feel sure exactly what is being demanded of us by others in terms of our response to their misfortunes.

And how do we stop our own personal histories from intruding in these responses? The deeper and more painful the events we are a witness to, the more likely it is that they will evoke some echo within us born of our own personal history, and thus that we may cast some shadow over our responses which distorts our perceptions and may make us act inappropriately. It is only too easy to let this personal patina shade our ability to respond with sensitivity to others' distress, and even the most balanced person may find themselves unable to detach their own personal history with its own scars and wounds from these responses.

To my patients, faced with some heavy blow of fate, I say, when asked that much-asked question, 'Why me?', that we can never know the answer to such a question, and thus to dwell on the reason for it is a waste of time. Instead, I say, we need to accept what is happening as a fate we have been handed, and thus as a task to fulfil. We may see some strands leading from our past actions to the present which may help to explain some aspects, but we may not be able to understand fully why we have been given this particular burden to bear. To take responsibility for the whole load may lead us too easily into assuming a corrosive level of guilt that only compounds the burden. If we have indeed done such wrong that we deserve this level of punishment, then the weight of this guilt may threaten to cripple us. How, then do we fit what can be viewed as the inequitable burdens some have been asked to bear within our overall view of human fate?

My Indian friend asked me incredulously one day, 'Why do you in the West expect to be happy? We just accept', and there is much in this approach to admire and learn from. How, though, do we accept, without becoming thereby passive, as though shrugging our shoulders in some gesture of resignation? There is surely some greater imperative here than a fatalistic passivity; some active responses have to be demanded of us if we are to have some goal to strive for. It seems to me that the deepest level of human existence represents a struggle of some kind, an attempt to change something in a more fruitful direction, the kind of transformation implicit in the idea that the kind of breakdown which tragic events can induce can, if approached creatively and positively, at the same time become a breakthrough, a breaking out from the past into some differently shaped future, whose shape we can determine by our actions. Any event then has the potential to move us forward in some way, just as the same event, if not approached creatively, can also pin us down as though trapping us in the past.

Tragic events, the raw unhappinesses which punctuate the smooth flow of life at different intervals for different people, can then assume a purpose hidden behind the sufferings they cause. They can force us to reposition ourselves in relation to our previous experiences, and in so doing bring about shifts in perspective which would otherwise not have occurred. The more radical this change in orientation, the greater can become the potential for inner development. It can provide what can be seen as a necessary jolt, like some painful electrical charge, jerking us to greater awareness.

And thus it seems to me appropriate that I should complete this book with an article I wrote some years ago about the death of a young patient of mine, which became for me, not, as I had expected, simply a tragic event, but much more importantly a transformative moment in my life, shaping much of my thinking about life and death and helping me to absorb this thinking into my future practice.

HEALING IN DEATH
Soul Door

Martine was a young patient of mine suffering from advanced cancer who was to die a year after we met.

A natural death, at the end of a full life, should not disturb us, for surely those who are old have had many a year to prepare themselves. But how are we to view the apparently appalling destiny of a young person dying early, and thus fighting a very different kind of battle? Unless we are compelled by illness or disaster, few of us pause to dwell upon the prospect of death. Thus we have had little practice in preparing ourselves for its approach. And when, as it did with my patient, Martine, death forces itself abruptly, in youth, it appears like some impenetrable barrier. The future, which we had taken for granted, now appears a prize torn from our grasp. No wonder there is bitterness and anger. Yet, as one Tibetan master has said, 'We are all going to die. Just some of us will die a little sooner than others.'

We can never stay neutral before death's advance, for it forces us out of a complacent acceptance of our right to be alive, making us redefine our attitude towards whatever time remains. It brings us face to face, often for the first time, with all those huge issues which touch upon the meaning of things. Everything becoming tinged with the hue of the impermanent, we can no longer measure things solely on a human time scale, but must set them against the wider backdrop of the eternal. There is much work to be done in assimilating this profound reorientation, and often, as with

Martine, so little time to do it in. Often, too, the extreme emotions which death arouses, like pressure upon some locked door, break open the protective defences we have spent a lifetime placing around ourselves. Death strips us naked, exposing our unresolved conflicts and demanding that they be dealt with, and never more so than in our close family relationships, for these have circumscribed and defined all aspects of our life. Now, as with all things death touches, they, too, are on the point of dissolving.

In the case of Martine, having spent much of her life in conflict with what she felt was a dominating and stifling mother, her anger grew so implacable shortly before she died that she forbade her mother to visit, defiantly leaving unopened all pleading letters. It would have been possible for me to stay neutral in this particular conflict, but our relationship had always been that of two people closely engaged in the most serious of all encounters, that of facing death. First we attempted together to halt its advance, then finally learned together to come to terms with its inevitability. I was very aware that Martine wanted help from me at many different levels. Obviously she wanted me to help her body heal, but equally urgently she seemed to be asking me, ever more insistently as death approached, for guidance for her spirit.

During the year of her treatment with me there had been many occasions when I had confronted her with what I felt was her self-indulgence in expressing resentment towards her family unhindered by any regard for the pain she was causing. I challenged her right to use her illness to absolve herself of any obligation towards others. Now, knowing how close to death she was, and what a terrible legacy of guilt she would leave her family if this conflict remained unresolved, I told her directly of my deep conviction that each of us has a duty to leave this world a better place than we found it. I asked her whether she felt her actions were contributing to this or not.

She told me not to lecture her because it was all too much for her. And I had to ask myself afterwards whether I had had any right to force the issue in this way, at this late stage. What if all I had done was to make things even worse? Then her sister rang to tell me that, the day after my visit, Martine had called her mother to her bedside, had kissed her, and told her that she was the person she had always loved the most. Three days later Martine was dead.

In all this, my role as acupuncturist overlapped with that of counsellor, and both were required to bring Martine some peace of mind as death approached. What I had said to her may have contributed to reconcile her with her mother, but acupuncture treatment had prepared the ground for change. This dual role of acupuncturist and counsellor raises the question of the aim of treatment. Brought up as we are in a culture in which medicine is restricted almost exclusively to treatment of the physical, it is tempting for us to measure success by purely physical criteria, asking ourselves whether the physical symptoms have disappeared or not. In the case of the milder forms of illness, physical criteria may not be a problem. But as severity increases so does the possibility, and at the most serious level, the probability, that physical symptoms will persist, despite our efforts. Do we then view treatment as a failure? Or must we turn to other criteria?

Acupuncturists accept three levels which make up the human being. First, there is the body, which we can touch and see. Then we delve deeper to reach the mind, which we can neither touch nor see, being that part of us which thinks and works things out, our intermediary between inner and outer being. And finally, at the deepest level of all, we come upon the spirit. Spirit is hidden so deep within that many in the West question its very existence. Yet is it so clearly there that we all understand what is meant by one person being 'full of spirit' and another 'dispirited'.

Once the body is damaged beyond repair, treatment of any kind at the physical level can do little more than palliate. Yet it is never too late, until the very moment of death, to extend healing to the mind and, in particular, to the profound needs of the spirit. Here we come to what is particularly relevant for the seriously ill, because as the body declines, our inner powers, nourished as they are by a different form of energy, can remain largely independent. Unhampered by physical limitations, the mind and spirit can roam in much wider pastures than those to which our body restricts us. The work we can do on our inner development knows no boundaries. And at this new level, mind, and above all spirit, lead the way, the mind working towards an understanding of the context in which to place illness, the spirit at last feeling at one with life's mysteries.

With severely ill or dying patients, I see my work as acupuncturist as helping them make that difficult transition from an assumption that the only hope lies in saving the body to a realization that there is a deeper form of survival. And it could be said that such an understanding puts them in touch with what is eternal within themselves.

Five element acupuncture is based upon the knowledge that each of us develops a special relationship with one of the five elements of which all life is composed. The balance of all the elements one with another constitutes health, their imbalance ill-health. But for each one of us there is a leader among the elements, I call it our guardian element, to whose demands we must listen if we are to fulfil the particular purpose our life demands. And each element has its own needs and weaknesses and strengths.

In Martine's case, the element that dominated her life was Fire, the element of relationship, of love and joy, of laughter and warmth, sheltering within itself the heart. And relationships, or rather their negative shadow, dominated her life. All the joyous outpourings towards others for which the

Fire element yearns had turned, in her, to a bitter refusal to relate to anybody, least of all to her family. Yet she could not escape the pull of these relationships, until, ironically and appropriately, her illness finally forced her back home. It was as though this illness, at one level a tragedy, on a deeper level became an instrument of forgiveness and thus of salvation.

Even though, by the end, treatment gave only the slightest respite to her body, it had grown increasingly effective at those other levels of mind and spirit. Thus, after each treatment until quite close to her death, she would say, 'I feel marvellous now.' And, although her body was invaded by tumours, to the very end she needed no painkillers. She even chided herself, remarkable woman that she was, for briefly accepting medication to ease vomiting. Apart from that, she allowed the needle to do its profound work. At its touch, that haunted and haunting look so often seen in the eyes of the dying, as though they see past us deep into the frightening unknown, was replaced, for however brief a time, by the serenity of a soul at peace.

Only one who has actually seen such transformation after acupuncture treatment can truly believe that change of this kind is possible. But her family and I observed it, and, perhaps, so too did the staff at the hospice, for her strength of spirit amazed them.

After Martine's death, her sister said to me, 'How can you say that there was any point to all her suffering? Perhaps you are fooling yourself that there was.' Perhaps. Yet, just before her death, we felt that the small hospice room was filled with the powerful presence of a spirit reaching far beyond Martine's now shrunken, almost irrelevant body. It was as though this body had become, no longer a shell, but a chrysalis from which her soul was slowly released, to speed who knows where?

None of us, except now Martine, can know what purpose her death and the manner of it has had for her. It certainly brought her clearly to face things she had avoided looking at before; and by the end, after much tumultuous heart-searching, it brought her to forgive those close to her, something she had strenuously resisted. It could be argued that the extreme emotion aroused by approaching death may sometimes be the only thing that enables us to confront what we have avoided. And if this is so, which I have come to believe, then there is purpose to such a death, for surely we should all die only when we have tied up loose ends and completed our life.

The possibility of such a purpose undoubtedly has relevance for Martine herself, but just as much for others coming into contact with death. No one who has sat by death's side emerges from such an awesome encounter untouched. The more apparently tragic that death, the greater the effect it must have upon all who witness it. In that, too, there may lie a purpose which only those who participate in such an event can fathom. In my own case, I know that it has been from Martine that I have learned the most in my attempt to find some perspective on death, perhaps because I have had to dig deep inside myself to struggle with my own horror at what seemed the waste of such a young life.

When the soul emerges strong from such a battle with death as Martine had to confront, death finds us, not crushed, but triumphant. How much more so this must hold true for those who have been chosen from among so many to die young.

Reprint of an article from the journal Meridians, *Winter 1994. Reprinted by kind permission of the Maryland University of Integrative Health, Maryland, USA, formerly the Tai Sophia Institute, www.muih.edu.*